Risk in Social Work Practice

The study of 'risk' in social work involves complex interplay between human behaviour, emotion, evidence of fact, professional values and organisational systems. This book brings together contributions from key social work researchers and theorists from the UK, USA, New Zealand and Italy, writing with a focus on aspects of risk within social work. It examines key debates concerning risk in contemporary social work practice, including ethical dilemmas, approaches to decision-making and the challenges of ignorance and errors. Contributions range from the perennial challenges of how one uses formal knowledge when assessing risk to emerging risks arising from the counterterrorism agenda. This book will enable practitioners, policy makers and researchers to appreciate the complexities of risk in different settings and apply this understanding to their own practice.

This book was originally published as a special issue of the *Journal of Social Work Practice*.

Andrew Whittaker is an Associate Professor of Social Work at London South Bank University, UK, where he is the Head of the Risk, Resilience and Expert Decision Making research group. His research focuses on child protection and the risks faced by young people in cities.

Brian Taylor is a Professor of Social Work at Ulster University, Coleraine, UK, where he leads the Decision, Assessment, Risk and Evidence Studies research cluster. He is the author of *Decision Making, Assessment and Risk in Social Work* (2017, 3rd ed) and *Understanding and Using Research in Social Work* (with Anne McGlade and Campbell Killick, 2015).

Risk in Social Work Practice

Current Issues

Edited by
Andrew Whittaker and Brian Taylor

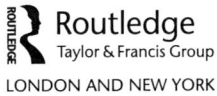
Routledge
Taylor & Francis Group

LONDON AND NEW YORK

First published 2019
by Routledge
2 Park Square, Milton Park, Abingdon, Oxon, OX14 4RN, UK

and by Routledge
52 Vanderbilt Avenue, New York, NY 10017

First issued in paperback 2020

Routledge is an imprint of the Taylor & Francis Group, an informa business

British Library Cataloguing-in-Publication Data
A catalogue record for this book is available from the British Library

ISBN 13: 978-0-367-58647-8 (pbk)
ISBN 13: 978-1-138-59995-6 (hbk)

Typeset in Perpetua
by codeMantra

Publisher's Note
The publisher accepts responsibility for any inconsistencies that may have arisen during the conversion of this book from journal articles to book chapters, namely the possible inclusion of journal terminology.

Disclaimer
Every effort has been made to contact copyright holders for their permission to reprint material in this book. The publishers would be grateful to hear from any copyright holder who is not here acknowledged and will undertake to rectify any errors or omissions in future editions of this book.

Contents

CONTENTS

Citation Information

The chapters in this book were originally published in the *Journal of Social Work Practice*, volume 31, issue 4 (December 2017). When citing this material, please use the original page numbering for each article, as follows:

Chapter 6

'Risk is King and Needs to Take a Backseat!' Can Social Workers' Experiences of Moral Injury Strengthen Practice?
Jane Fenton and Timothy B. Kelly
Journal of Social Work Practice, volume 31, issue 4 (December 2017) pp. 461–476

Chapter 7

A Risky Time for Muslim Families: Professionalised Counter-Radicalisation Networks
Tony Stanley, Surinder Guru and Vicki Coppock
Journal of Social Work Practice, volume 31, issue 4 (December 2017) pp. 477–490

Chapter 8

Reflective Practice, Risk and Mistakes in Social Work
Alessandro Sicora
Journal of Social Work Practice, volume 31, issue 4 (December 2017) pp. 491–502

For any permission-related enquiries please visit:
http://www.tandfonline.com/page/help/permissions

Notes on Contributors

Laura L. Cook is a Lecturer in the School of Social Work at the University of East Anglia, Norwich, UK. Her research focuses on decision-making in social work, particularly the role of emotion in professional judgement.

Vicki Coppock is a Professor of Childhood Studies and Mental Health in the Department of Social Sciences at Edge Hill University, Ormskirk, UK. Her research focuses on critical social scientific analysis of theory, state policy and professional practice in childhood and youth, with a particular emphasis on asserting a positive human rights agenda for children and young people in distress or 'trouble'.

Jane Fenton is a Senior Lecturer and the Head of Taught Postgraduate Studies at the University of Dundee, UK. Her research interests include the disconnect between social work values and practice and social justice.

Eileen Gambrill is a Professor of the graduate school of the School of Social Welfare at the University of California, Berkeley, USA. Her research interests include ethics and decision-making in the helping professions focusing on the integration of evidentiary and ethical concerns, and propaganda in the helping professions.

Surinder Guru teaches on the Social Work programs in the Department of Social Work and Social Care at the University of Birmingham, UK. Her current research focuses on the impact of counterterrorism policies on the families and communities and role of social work interventions.

Peter Hall is a Senior Lecturer in the Social Work BA (Hons) Social Work programme in the Department of Psychology, Sociology and Social Work at the University of Suffolk, Ipswich, UK, and is an External Examiner for the University of Leeds, UK, and Northumbria University, Newcastle upon Tyne, UK.

Mark Hardy is a Senior Lecturer in Social Work at the University of York, UK. He has published widely on the role of knowledge in practice. He is the editor of the four-volume *SAGE Major Work on Social Work Research* (2015, with Jeanne Marsh and Ian Shaw) and of *Mental Health Social Work: The Art and Science of Practice* (forthcoming, with Martin Webber).

Emily Keddell is a Senior Lecturer in Social Work at the University of Otago, Dunedin, New Zealand. Her research interests include understanding risk, decision-making and inequalities in child welfare.

NOTES ON CONTRIBUTORS

Timothy B. Kelly is a Professor of Social Work and Dean of the School of Education and Social Work at the University of Dundee, UK. His research interests include group work, the health and social care needs of older people and their carers and social work ethics.

Alessandro Sicora is an Associate Professor of Social Work at University of Trento, Italy, and Research Associate of the Department of Social Work at the Stellenbosch University, South Africa. His research interests include methods of social work, comparative social policy, reflexive practice, professional mistakes and aggression against social workers.

Tony Stanley is a Chief Social Worker for Birmingham City Council, UK. He is the professional lead for quality social work and improving practice for vulnerable children and their families. He is researching social workers' constructions of 'family' in radicalisation risk cases.

Brian Taylor is a Professor of Social Work at Ulster University, Coleraine, UK, where he leads the Decision, Assessment, Risk and Evidence Studies research cluster. He is the author of *Decision Making, Assessment and Risk in Social Work* (2013) and *Understanding and Using Research in Social Work* (with Anne McGlade and Campbell Killick, 2015).

Andrew Whittaker is an Associate Professor of Social Work at London South Bank University, UK, where he is the Head of the Risk, Resilience and Expert Decision Making research group. His research focuses on child protection and the risks faced by young people in cities.

Andrew Whittaker and Brian Taylor

INTRODUCTION

Understanding Risk in Social Work

Welcome to this special issue of the Journal of Social Work Practice on *risk in social work*. *Risk* is often defined in terms of the probability of harm occurring (Gigerenzer 2014); although in social work practice, the concept is far more multi-faceted. The profession is concerned with the seriousness of (i.e. negative value placed on) the particular harm as well as its likelihood. When we consider 'risky situations' in terms of making decisions, we are often considering both potential gains (with both their value and their likelihood) as well as the possible harms in some way or other (Taylor 2017a). Consideration of future situations raises the complex domain of deciding about preventive actions to reduce the possibility or seriousness of harm. And then there are the emotions such as *wariness of lurking conflict* (Taylor 2006), anxiety, fear and courage – familiar subject matter to readers of this journal – which may be an intrinsic part of such 'risk work' within professional practice. To give added complexity, we must consider also the organisational system aspects, such as the assessment and management of risk, which interweaves with the professional tasks (Taylor et al. 2015). Working in 'risk averse' organisations and within a wider societal culture of blame are challenges that practitioners must work with everyday (Cooper & Whittaker 2014; Whittaker 2011; Whittaker & Havard 2016). The study of 'risk' in social work is a fundamental topic of interest to this journal, where there is a complex interplay between human behaviour, emotion, evidence of fact, professional values and organisational systems. This special issue includes articles from esteemed social work researchers and theorists from around the globe, writing with a focus on aspects of risk within social work. We are delighted to welcome their contributions!

Eileen Gambrill from the USA writes about: *avoidable ignorance and the ethics of risk in child welfare*. This scholarly piece by a world-renowned social work academic highlights the moral demand for greater openness in providing information to clients about the outcomes of services so that informed choices may be made. The article is based on a systemic view of risk to children and families, and draws links between appraising risk and the use of client decision aids.

The article by Mark Hardy (England) is titled: *in defence of actuarialism: interrogating the logic of risk in social work practice*. He discusses concerns that an emphasis on 'risk' in social work might tend to focus on individual pathology and neglect consideration of the social environment. This provides a context for his study of practitioner decision-making which challenged this critique. The study data suggest that sometimes practitioners have greater concerns than the facts warrant. The tendency to 'risk aversion' seems to be more a feature of working environments in which fear of blame is a concern, rather than being a function of the use of actuarial assessment tools. Emotion seems to over-ride objective statistical calculation leading to risk-averse practice. The use of robust assessment tools may provide a necessary check and balance in emotionally demanding work.

Emily Keddell presents the results of a rigorous study set in New Zealand which compares: *risk-averse and risk-friendly practitioners in child welfare decision-making*. Attitudes of practitioners to risk issues were studied using vignettes. The study found that non-governmental social workers were more inclined to be risk-averse by comparison with statutory child welfare workers. Risk-averse practitioners, who rated the severity of the abuse higher than the risk-friendly group, estimated more harm to children over time if there was no intervention even though both groups described the problems experienced by the vignette family using similar constructs and with similar causal explanations of the behaviours. The use of the term 'risk-friendly' in the article acknowledges the negative cultural connotations that can exist around the term 'risk-taking', even whilst professionals acknowledge that risk-aversion may not always be the best decision choice. One conclusion of the study is that practitioners may differ in terms of orientation between a 'developmental-lifespan' focus compared to a 'presenting-welfare-needs' focus, leading to a different conceptualisation and weighting of risk factors.

There are three articles in this issue that focus on emotional aspects of 'risk work' in professional practice. Laura Cook (England) seeks to make sense of initial home visits in terms of: *the role of intuition in child and family social workers' assessments of risk*. Practitioners reported that intuitions during their first encounter with the family were an important source of information for assessment of risk. Emotional responses such as 'niggles' and 'gut feelings' sensitised them to potentially important information before it was processed rationally. The study identifies five heuristics (human judgement shortcuts; see Taylor 2017b) used by social workers to assess risk during the initial encounter, providing a connection between 'risk-work' and professional judgement tasks.

Peter Hall (England) writes on: *Mental Health Act assessments: professional narratives on alternatives to hospital admission*. He draws on interviews with professionals involved with Mental Health Act assessments to illustrate concepts of decision-making, professional boundaries and models of these assessments, which are explored as a means of understanding outcomes to Mental Health Act assessments.

Jane Fenton and Timothy Kelly (Scotland) focus on *social workers' experiences of moral injury* using a concept developed to refer to shame and guilt disturbances experienced by combat veterans, manifesting with some of the symptoms of post-traumatic stress disorder. Their study found that the more risk averse an agency is, the more ethical stress was experienced by workers. Qualitative data from the study is integrated with concepts of 'moral injury' in terms of situations where social workers perpetrate, fail to prevent or witness acts that contravene their moral code. They propose that for social workers to operate in a healthy and service-user-driven manner, they must retain the ability and flexibility to engage in reflection and responsive practice.

Although many of the issues facing social workers have been broadly similar for decades, the next article – by Tony Stanley, Surinder Guru and Vicki Coppock (England) – illustrates a modern challenge: the role of social workers in relation to: 'counter-radicalisation networks'. The context is new statutory responsibilities placed on professionals in England to pay: 'due regard to preventing terrorism'.

This duty seems to have contributed to a shifting of social work practice and decision-making from the fields of advocacy and promotion of ethics, justice and human rights, towards risk work more analogous to that of security services. Based on case study material, the article discusses issues for social workers engaged in anticipatory risk work, working in a pre-crime space in an effort to prevent terrorist atrocities.

The final article in this issue is by Alessandro Sicora from Italy. Alessandro focuses on: *reflective practice, risk and mistakes in social work*. His paper develops further some risk concepts outlined in his recent book (Sicora 2017). He highlights a wide range of aspects from the emotional experience of 'being wrong' to organisational systems for error prevention and for highlighting latent errors. He proposes that 'reasonable' professional decision-making can be developed through appropriate reflective practice opportunities. This provides a positive and hopeful complement to articles that necessarily deal with the many difficult and painful issues of possible harm to people that we conceptualise as 'risk'.

These articles present a welcome and interesting range of study findings and perspectives on risk in social work. However, the topic of 'risk' in social work requires further development, despite the proliferation of sociological literature on the one hand, and the organisation material on 'managing risks' on the other. Our own professional social work approach to risk is only slowly emerging, through ideas in articles such as these. Our challenge is to integrate useful ideas from other fields – including communication studies, health care, law, military studies, organisational science, psychology and sociology – and develop our own conceptualisation suited to our professional role.

When the call went out for this special issue, abstracts were invited that related to both decision-making and risk. In the event, the number of high-quality abstracts received was such that the journal editors decided to allow two special issues: this one focusing more on risk, and one next year focusing on professional judgement and decision-making. So, journal readers have a second special issue to look forward to! However, the topics of risk and decision-making are closely linked such that both special issues will have relevance to both topics to some extent.

One reason for the strong response to the abstract call is key networks that are growing on this topic area. Firstly, the *Decisions, Assessment, Risk and Evidence in Social Work* (DARE) biennial conference near Belfast, Northern Ireland has now been running since 2010 (www.ulster.ac.uk/dare). The last (2016) conference attracted over 120 participants from 12 countries; the next conference is planned for July 2018. Secondly, the *Decisions, Assessment and Risk Special Interest Group* (DARSIG) of the *European Social Work Research Association* (ESWRA) (Taylor & Sharland 2015) was formed in 2014 (Taylor et al. 2017). DARSIG is in its early stages of development, but already includes over 30 members from about 15 countries. Some key areas for research and development on risk in social work have been identified by the group, including: the influence of organisational and national cultures on understandings of 'risk'; the place of consequences as well as likelihoods in judging risk; models of how potential benefits are weighed against possible harm; how 'big data' might inform our understanding of risk factors; linking risk with strengths and mitigating factors; risk within social work assessment; the interface between risk and preventive services; and developing effective methods of communicating risk with numbers, words or visual means. Readers interested in the topic of risk in social work are warmly invited, of course, to attend the DARE conference or to join DARSIG through the ESWRA website (http://www. eswra.org/).

If you are pursuing research, teaching or development of management or practice on some dimension of risk in social work, we would like to encourage you in your endeavours. But even if your interest is limited to reading this journal, we hope that you enjoy these stimulating articles.

References

Cooper, A., & Whittaker, A. (2014). History as tragedy, never as farce: Tracing the long cultural narrative of child protection in England. *Journal of Social Work Practice, 28*(3), 251–266.

Gigerenzer, G. (2014). *Risk savvy: How to make good decisions*. New York, NY: Penguin.

Sicora, A. (2017). *Reflective practice and learning from mistakes in social work*. Bristol: Policy Press.

Taylor, B. J. (2006). Risk management paradigms in health and social services for professional decision making on the long-term care of older people. *British Journal of Social Work, 36*(8), 1411–1429.

Taylor, B. J. (2017a). *Decision making, assessment and risk in social work* (3rd ed.). London: Sage.

Taylor, B. J. (2017b). Heuristics in professional judgement: A psycho-social rationality model. *British Journal of Social Work, 47*(4), 1043–1060.

Taylor, B. J., Killick, C., & McGlade, A. (2015). *Understanding and using research in social work*. London: Sage.

Taylor, B. J., & Sharland, E. (2015). The creation of the European social work research association. *Research on Social Work Practice, 25*(5), 623–627.

Taylor, B.J., Killick, C., Bertotti, T., Enosh, G., Gautschi, J., Hietamäki, J., Sicora, A. & Whittaker A. (2017) European Social Work Research Association SIG to study decisions, assessment and risk. *Journal of Evidence-Informed Social Work*, 15(1), 82–94. doi:10.1080/23761407.2017.1394244

Whittaker, A. (2011). Social defences and organisational culture in a local authority child protection setting: Challenges for the Munro Review? *Journal of Social Work Practice, 25*(4), 481–495.

Whittaker, A., & Havard, T. (2016). Defensive practice as 'fear-based' practice: Social work's open secret? *British Journal of Social Work, 46*(5), 1158–1174.

Eileen Gambrill

AVOIDABLE IGNORANCE AND THE ETHICS OF RISK IN CHILD WELFARE

Sources of risk to children include far more than risk of harm to children from biological parents. Key opportunities to reveal and decrease avoidable ignorance that contribute to avoidable risk to children and families have been neglected such as clearly describing the evidentiary status of services provided and outcomes attained. A systemic view of risk requires attention to faulty assessment, referral to agencies that offer ineffective programs, failure to monitor outcomes and the quality of the social worker-client relationship on an ongoing basis, dysfunctional organizational arrangements, and failure to involve clients as informed participants. An examination of the websites of child welfare agencies in the San Francisco Bay Area revealed that not one offered information that would enable informed decision making. Education programs may fail to help students to acquire skills in the process of evidence-informed practice. Based on a systemic view of risk, an agenda to decrease avoidable ignorance that contributes to avoidable risks to children and families is suggested emphasizing informed consent obligations. This includes increasing transparency regarding what is done to what effect including professional education and welcoming criticism of practices and policies and related claims. Reasons for failure to reveal and decrease such ignorance are explored including economic interests in the adoption and child welfare services industry.

Decision-making is key in the helping professions and a rich literature is available that can guide decisions, including research regarding risk – kinds, sources and obstacles to revealing, understanding and reducing (e.g. Gigerenzer 2014; Taylor 2013; Vincent 2010). Consideration of risk involves: (1) selection of risks to focus on; (2) care with which related factors and consequences are described guided by relevant research and theory; (3) resources devoted to exploring how to minimise risk; (4) who and how to involve in decision-making; (5) selection of assessment and intervention methods designed to minimise risk; (6) clarity and relevance with which evaluation of results are explored; and (7) degree of transparency to all involved parties regarding criteria used to make decisions and outcomes achieved. Decisions made by child welfare staff include whether to investigate reports of abuse and/or neglect, how to estimate risk to children, whether to remove a child from his or her home, what services to purchase and what criteria to rely on when doing so, when to close a case, how often to

Part of this paper is based on a presentation at a conference on "Risk in Social Services and Its Consequences." Bath, England, 9/24/03.

visit a home, and when to return a child to parents. Other decisions concern whether to honour ethical (and/or) legal requirements such as informed consent, kind of staff training to provide, whether to seek out and try to minimise avoidable errors, whether to implement and act on the results of a user-friendly complaint system, and what kind of organisational cultures to encourage.

Risks differ in their source, kind, timing, duration, probability, probability of harm and whom they affect. They differ in how much control we have over them and in our beliefs about who is responsible for them. They may be avoidable or unavoidable. Ignorance, both unavoidable and chosen, as well as knowledge, is integral to exploring each of these dimensions. We know what many risks are in child welfare and that some are avoidable or can be minimised such as provision of ineffective services. Staff in child protective agencies are daily confronted by heart rending circumstances with insufficient resources to address them. They are often ill-trained and overburdened. Risk in child welfare includes possible harm as a result of lost opportunities to help children and families (e.g. referring clients to agencies that provide poor quality service). Problems and related harms in the child welfare system have been clear for some time, including dysfunctional recording systems, inappropriate prescription of psychotropic medication for children in foster care (e.g. Allen 2015; Bartholet 1999) and institutional abuse (e.g. New Jersey Office of the Child Advocate 2008). Indeed, so little momentum has been achieved in decreasing avoidable risks to children and families that we must explore why. Is this because of the vulnerability of families involved in the child welfare system (e.g. many are poor)?

The context: a systemic view of risk

Sources of risk to children and families include far more than risk of harm to children from biological parents. Discovering opportunities to enhance the quality of care for children and families requires attention to the context of care as many have noted (e.g. Gambrill & Shlonsky 2001; Wulczyn et al. 2010). A key source of avoidable risk to children and families stems from failure to use a systemic approach to risk in which avoidable ignorance that contributes to avoidable risks to children and families is revealed and addressed. A systemic view of risk is needed to discover leverage points for minimising avoidable risks. Characteristics of naturalistic decision-making include ill-structured problems, uncertain changing environments, multiple players, shifting, ill-defined, competing goals, action/feedback loops (not one-shot decisions) and time pressures (Klein 2015). According to IBISWorld.com the Adoption and Child Welfare Services Industry is a 14.3 billion dollar industry with a projected annual growth of 1.5%. Millions of people earn their living in this industry. Related organisations and industries spend money to shape beliefs and actions in ways that favour their interests. Involved parties include governmental officials, administrators, supervisors, those who provide services, educators, researchers and editorial boards of journals. Political, social and economic interests contribute to identifying a given situation, person, characteristic or consequence as a risk. We emphasise some risks and ignore others (Slovic 2010). Some argue that risks are created to allow agents of the government to take coercive action against those labelled as at risk or as a risk to others (Szasz 1994). Risk is big business. Pharmaceutical companies forward the creation of risks and promote medications to reduce them (e.g. Angel 2011). Hundreds of behaviours are framed as brain diseases requiring medication (Schwarz 2016). Concerns about increasing privatisation of services have long been raised.

The ethics of risk

Each profession has a code of ethics that contains prescriptions (what we should do – as provide effective services to clients), as well as proscriptions (what we should not do – harm clients). Ethical obligations require professionals to be conversant with research related to key decisions and to meet obligations for informed consent (e. g, National Association of Social Workers 2008). The ethics of risk involves considering the benefits and harms of different ways in which risk is viewed and handled. For example, is it ethical to refer clients to agencies that do not provide effective services and do not involve clients as informed participants? Is it ethical to expect staff to do certain tasks but not provide the resources needed? A systemic view of risk illustrates that the ethics of risk is both a personal as well as a political matter. (See prior discussion of context.) It is a personal matter because we each make choices about how critically to think about our decisions including how they affect others. The ethics of risk highlights our obligation to be informed about avoidable risks and related causes, including unexplained variations in practices. It highlights our obligation to accurately assess both personal and objective ignorance related to risks to children and families and to take action to decrease avoidable risks including miminizing poor excuses for avoidable ignorance.

Avoidable ignorance as a key contributor to avoidable risk

There are many kinds and causes of ignorance including clashes between professional (to keep a job) and client interests (blow the whistle on harmful practices). A lens of ignorance invites us to ask: "What's missing?"; "What important questions remain unanswered?" "What are important uncertainties?" Ignoring vital information is often carefully planned and maintained; it is strategic (McGoey 2012). In child welfare, our guard may be down for deception – who would hinder policies and practices that help children and families? The field of agnotology, also referred to as the sociology of ignorance, highlights the social construction of ignorance, for example by the creation of doubt and censorship. Strategic ignorance is an asset. For example, it helps regulating agencies to avoid carrying out their key functions (McGoey 2007). The term "forbidden knowledge" refers to "Knowledge that is too sensitive, dangerous, or taboo to produce" (Kempner 2015, p.77), and I would add, reveal. This may be hidden in many ways – censorship, confusion, distortion and fabrication, key propaganda strategies (Gambrill 2012a). There may be a conspiracy of silence (Zerubavel 2006).

Professional education programmes, the professional literature, governmental accountability requirements and administrative policies and practices influence what is shared and what is not. Ignorance may be deliberately chosen (maintenance of known unknowns) such as the horrible conditions in which many children live, so removing responsibility for doing something about it. (See description of "devices of denial" in Ash 2016). Socially constructed ignorance influences risk to children and families in many ways including making decisions based on inaccurate claims about the effectiveness of assessment, intervention and/or evaluation methods. There are increasing revelations of bogus claims in the peer-reviewed literature, including systematic reviews (Ioannidis, 2005, 2016). Whenever money is involved, transparency of what is done to what effect is an uphill battle. Indeed, I recently shared with a child welfare researcher that I could not find one child welfare agency in the San Francisco Bay Area which clearly described the evidentiary status of services used and the fidelity with which they were implemented on its website. Her response was "Who would do that?"

Examples of avoidable ignorance that increases risk to children and families

Viewing practice and policy in child welfare through a lens of avoidable ignorance highlights interrelated sources of avoidable risks to children and families.

Failure to involve clients as informed participants

The Code of Ethics of the National Association of Social Workers (2008) in the United States states that:

> Social workers should use clear and understandable language to inform clients of the purpose of the services, risks related to the services, limits to services because of the requirements of a third-party payer, relevant costs, reasonable alternatives, clients' right to refuse or withdraw consent, and the time frame covered by the consent. Social workers should provide clients with an opportunity to ask questions.

Informed consent involves a process in which there are many opportunities to honour-related actions. Self-determination is integrally related to informed consent. What percentage of clients are accurately informed about risks and benefits of services provided? My students typically omit obligations to share information about risks and benefits of well-argued alternatives.

Only in recent years has shared decision-making been actively pursued in medicine. This refers to collaborative, deliberative, decision-making involving open, honest, empathic information sharing (Elwyn, Edwards, & Thompson 2016). Review of information offered to patients reveals most to be misleading (Gigerenzer & Gray 2011). Child welfare clients are typically not informed regarding the competency of the professionals they are required to see. Examination of the websites of many services to which child welfare clients are referred in the Bay Area shows that none clearly describes the evidentiary status of programmes, outcomes attained and information regarding competencies of staff to provide them. Lists of resources used are given on websites of Departments of Children and Family Services with no information that would allow a user of these services to make an informed decision about their use (e.g. Purchase of Service Directory (2014) for Hawaii). Vagueness is a key source of avoidable ignorance that may pose unnecessary risks to children and parents and violates informed consent requirements. There is a lack of transparency that violates ethical obligations to clients.

If clients are referred to ineffective programmes (e.g. parent training, substance abuse) and are not informed about this, they lose opportunities to discover whether they can attain required outcomes as a result of effective programmes and so acquire or maintain custody of their children. Children may lose opportunities to continue living with their parents. Children may be returned to dangerous situations. Failure to attend to the evidentiary status of programmes to which clients are referred and the fidelity with which they are offered makes social workers complicit in maintaining funding for poor programmes. Obligations regarding informed consent are not mentioned in articles promoting better service planning. It may be mentioned but not clarified. It seems to be a taboo topic.

Transparency is integral to informed consent. Informed consent requires sharing ignorance (for example, lack of information regarding the effectiveness of interventions), as well as knowledge. It requires accurate description of "well informed uncertainties" (Chalmers 2004). It requires sharing the track record of service providers to whom clients are referred in achieving hoped-for outcomes (Entwistle, Sheldon, Sowden, & Watt 1998). Failure to involve clients as informed participants contributes to risk in many ways. Indeed, it could be argued that honouring this ethical mandate would entail addressing most sources of avoidable ignorance that contribute to avoidable risk to children and families. It would require transparency of what is done to what effect and taking corrective action based on lapses discovered.

Objections and counterarguments to involving clients as informed participants including appeals to good intentions reflect avoidable ignorance and the need for advocacy.

Clients will not understand

This objection ignores developments in enhancing health literacy among clients as well as professionals (e.g. Perrenoud, Velonaki, Bodenmann, & Ramelet 2015).

Clients are not voluntary

Coercion does not remove informed consent obligations. Related opportunities include inviting clients to ask questions, informing clients about the evidentiary status of recommended services and alternatives (e.g. via user-friendly client decision aids, for example regarding parent-training programmes), and informing clients about possible consequences depending on their participation and/or attainment of certain objectives.

This will discourage client participation and decrease placebo effects

If participation would result in harm, *should* clients participate? It may be argued that accurately informing clients will compromise hope. The evidentiary status of services should be shared with clients in the context of a supportive relationship. Potential negative consequences of relying on placebo effects should be considered, such as increasing or maintaining dependency on unneeded services.

Clients don't want to know

Clients are obligated to share the burden of making decisions, especially when children are involved. The fact that information is not used does not remove the obligation to provide it. Parents have an ethical obligation to be informed about risks to their children including risk of being referred to ineffective programmes.

It takes too much time

Information can be provided via client decision aids on user-friendly websites and in brochures that would enable clients to inform themselves on their own time (Elwyn et al. 2016).

Staff are uninformed so cannot inform clients

Staff may protest that they do not have time to be informed about the evidentiary status of services they offer and/or that other agencies offer. Their objections may be realistic and require advocacy to address-related factors. Agencies from which services are purchased should be required to provide this information.

No effective services are available

In child protective settings, even if parents are told that a service is unlikely to be helpful, they may have to participate or their children will be taken away or not be returned. This does not remove the ethical obligation to accurately inform them about the evidentiary status of services.

Appeal to standard of care

Involving clients as informed participants is more the exception than the rule. Here again we see the necessity of advocacy (see later discussion).

Avoidable ignorance regarding quality of services and outcomes

What percentage of children are protected from further harm? What percentage thrive? Exactly what do involved staff have to know (content knowledge) and do (procedural knowledge) to provide competent help? The greater the cultural differences between staff and clients, the greater may be the need for related knowledge and resources to negotiate them. Unanswered questions include: What variations occur and do these reveal inequities such as different quality services in different areas? What percentage of staff offer high levels of common factors such as warmth and empathy that contribute to positive outcomes (Wampold & Imel 2015) as reflected in ongoing feedback (Lambert 2010; Miller, Hubble, Chow, & Seidel 2015)? Are staff well-informed regarding the science of behaviour (Thyer 2005)? What percentage of decisions are well reasoned (e.g. avoid influence of common biases and detect harmful trajectories (Gambrill 2012b)? What percentage of referrals result in hoped-for outcomes? Barth et al. (2005) state that there are no accurate estimates of how many parents "receive a reasonable dose of parent training ... or what the outcome might be" (p. 148). In what percentage of cases is monitoring arranged that protects children from harm? In what percentage of cases is progress accurately monitored in a timely manner that guides intervention planning? Are booster sessions provided when needed?

Avoidable ignorance due to use of inaccurate risk and safety assessment

Does an agency use the most predictive risk and safety assessment methods? Is risk assessment followed by an individualised assessment?

Avoidable ignorance concerning decision-making and expertise

Lack of knowledge and related skills regarding decision-making and how expertise is developed and maintained may result in harms that could have been avoided. Situation awareness involving pattern recognition is important (Klein 2015) including revising assessments as needed and arranging for feedback regarding outcome. Methodological challenges include definitional dilemmas (what is child abuse or child neglect?), lack of reliability and validity of measures (e.g. risk assessment), changes in risk over time, and problems in predicting for individuals (Gambrill & Shlonsky 2000). Cultivation and maintenance of expertise requires ongoing practice offering corrective feedback (Ericsson 2015; Rousmaniere et al. 2017). Poor communication among staff and between clients and helpers contributes to avoidable risk, as does the play of cognitive and affective biases including confirmation biases, hindsight bias, outcome bias and availability biases (Gambrill 2012b; Spratt, Devaney, & Hayes 2015). Ignorance concerning concepts such as false positive, false negative rate, cost-benefit ratio, absolute and relative risk may contribute to poor decisions (e.g. Gigerenzer 2014). Literature on risk describes many ways in which we may be led astray in estimating risk including how a problem is framed. Values, knowledge and skills involved in critical thinking that contribute to making informed decisions may be absent (Gambrill & Gibbs 2017). Little systematic attention has been paid to the identification of errors in child welfare such as incorrect framing of problems. Failure to identify errors, explore related causes and take remedial steps is an avoidable source of ignorance that may contribute to risk to children and families. Are staff and client decision aids used drawing on developments in other professions (e.g. Elwyn et al. 2016; Sheehan & Sherman 2012)?

Avoidable ignorance due to professional education programmes

What percentage of professional education programmes provide knowledge, skills and values in critical thinking that contribute to honouring the ethics of risk including developing skills, knowledge and values needed for life-long learning? Critiques of programmes in the United States are not encouraging (e.g. Stoesz, Karger, & Carrilio 2010). Each professional education programme, including continuing education programmes, may reflect a unique profile of avoidable ignorance, including promotion of false knowledge (Munz 1985). Such programmes may fail to provide a systemic understanding of risk and how to accurately estimate risk, and avoid common biases in making decisions. Those who raise questions may be punished rather than thanked, contributing to avoidable ignorance.

Avoidable ignorance concerning the process of evidence-based practice

The original vision of evidence-based practice was of a five-step process designed to help practitioners and clients to make informed decisions – informed about the degree of uncertainty surrounding those decisions (Sackett, Richardson, Rosenberg, & Haynes 1997). This process is often ignored in discussions of evidence-based practices (EBPs) and evidence-based interventions (EBIs). The EBIs and EBPs initiatives are top down initiatives; researchers and policy-makers advise or tell practitioners what to do. Promotion of EBPs and EBIs may discourage appropriate questioning of recommendations, based for example on variations in client circumstances and characteristics including cultural differences and concerns about conflicts of interests in guideline development (e.g. Cosgrove, Bursztajn, Erlich, Wheeler, & Shaughnessy 2013).

Avoidable ignorance regarding the flawed nature of the professional literature

Ignorance regarding the flawed nature of the professional literature impedes informed decisions. The peer-reviewed literature is replete with inflated claims of effectiveness that may provide misleading directions (e.g. Ioannidis 2005, 2016) and often hides controversies concerning problem framing (e.g. Rapley, Moncrieff, & Dillon 2011). Most publications in child welfare promoting use of EBPs and EBIs ignore this literature. Critical appraisal shows that websites and registries listing EBPs and EBIs may ignore conflicts of interests and minimal evidence in promotion of EBPs (Gorman 2017).

Avoidable ignorance due to failure to harvest questions

Failure to gather questions from clients and staff and seek answers to them is another source of avoidable risk. What are clients' and social workers' unanswered questions? Are these used to inform research priorities?

Avoidable ignorance regarding fraud and corruption that increases risk

Fraudulent claims about the effectiveness of interventions may result in overlooking effective methods or being harmed. Legal aspects of fraud include: (1) misrepresentation of a material fact; (2) knowledge of the falsity of the misrepresentation or ignorance of the truth; (3) intent; (4) acting on the misrepresentation; and (5) damage to the victim (*The Free Dictionary*). Institutional corruption occurs "when there is a systematic and strategic influence which is legal or even currently ethical, that undermines the institution's effectiveness by diverting it from its purpose or weakening its ability to achieve its purpose …" (Lessig 2013, p.553). Corruption, fraud, quackery and the propaganda ploys used in their service, compromise informed consent. Avoidable risks continue because of failing to blow the whistle on such practices. Instances of incompetence, corruption and fraud in child welfare are usually brought to our attention by reporters and bloggers. For example, National Mentor Holdings, Inc. provides foster homes for at-risk children in the United States. Roston (2015) reported that it is a $1.2 billion company with a history of violations. (See also Roston & Singer-Vine 2015).

Avoidable ignorance created by governmental sources and related funding patterns

Grandiose expectations (that no child be harmed) may encourage hiding rather than seeking out and trying to understand risks and their causes and how to minimise them. Governmental agencies are complicit in failing to require the transparent accountability needed to reveal avoidable risks to children and their families. Such agencies are often named as defendants in wrongful death lawsuits regarding children in care (Pollack & Popham 2009). Such agencies should take a much more active role in revealing and changing policies and practices that harm clients.

Avoidable ignorance resulting from organisational practices and policies

Risk management programmes may concentrate on protecting staff from malpractice suits rather than protecting children from harm. Services may be compromised by flawed information management systems (Obradovic 2011). (See also discussions of managerialism and privatisation in child welfare.) Poor quality supervision may contribute to avoidable risks. Administrators may be unresponsive to staff stress and fatigue. Agency cultures may not support constructive criticism of practices and policies.

Avoidable ignorance created by personal obstacles

Lack of self-knowledge may contribute to poor decisions (e.g. overconfidence; Dunning, Heath, & Suls 2004). We each have an ethics of risk reflected, for example in how carefully we examine our assumptions. The choices we make reflect our personal ethics of risk, including how we respond to dysfunctional organisational practices. A common reaction I see among child welfare workers is one of powerlessness. There is a feeling of helplessness. Resignation in response to unsupportive work environments is not ethically acceptable if it interferes with pursuit of needed changes to help clients. Self-deception, such as incorrectly assuming services are effective, may create avoidable risk to clients; there is thus an ethics of self-deception.

The continuing fight for transparency: ethical obligations as a guide

Current views of risk are incomplete – they overlook risks to parents and children of not being involved as *informed* participants. Transparency is the enemy of those who benefit from obscurity. Obscuring the quality of services and outcomes attained reflects a strategic use of avoidable ignorance that maintains dysfunctional practices and policies that harm children and families. Vagueness hides daily indignities and harms such as continuing to live in rat-infested apartments because of failure to expose landlords who ignore violations. Honouring informed consent obligations would have a cascade effect in terms of need to gather and share required information describing what is done to what effect in all contexts including gaps between current practices and policies and what is most likely to help children and families. Professional codes of ethics provide the mandate and should provide the courage to seek transparency. Ethical obligations require placing the protection of clients first in conflicts with professional and bureaucratic interests. Professionals have an ethical obligation to recognise how ignorance, both personal and objective, contributes to avoidable risks to children and families and to take steps to minimise this.

An agenda for change

In the face of avoidable risks to clients we could do nothing, complain or work together with others to change things. The ethics of risk requires pursuit of the third option. Honouring ethical obligations for informed consent and competence would require all players in the system to clearly describe what is done to what effect.

Welcome criticism in all venues

The ethics of risk calls for recognising faulty arguments and questioning claims about what may help or harm clients. Critical thinking values, skills and knowledge including critical appraisal of different kinds of research is integral to honouring the ethics of risk (Gambrill & Gibbs 2017).

Create facilitating cultures in organisations

Developing and maintaining practices and policies that contribute to quality services (those that are effective in achieving hoped-for outcomes) require learning cultures in which staff continue to enhance their skills via feedback regarding the outcomes of decisions. Raising critical questions may not be welcome in authoritarian environments. Obstacles to acting on the ethics of risk include being fired, loss of promotion or being shunned as a troublemaker. This highlights the importance of creating organisational cultures that encourage systemic attention to ethical issues related to risk. Changes in policies and practices should not merely offer an illusion of improvement. Hoped-for conduct regarding the ethics of risk can only flower in a climate in which all parties are encouraged to think critically about all sources of risk and to act to reduce risk – one in which staff are encouraged to expose practices and policies that pose avoidable risks to children and parents – one in which effective skills in argumentation are encouraged (Walton 2015).

Make better use of technology

Agency administrators and those who fund agencies have an obligation to provide information management systems that contribute to quality services. We should take advantage of staff and client decision aids (e.g. Elwyn et al. 2016). Apps on smartphones can be used to remind staff about obligations to accurately inform clients about uncertainties related to decisions. Both outcome and process feedback from clients after each meeting should be gathered to maximise attainment of hoped-for outcomes (Miller et al. 2015).

Address-related lapses on the part of professional schools and continuing education programmes

Professional education programmes should take a more active role in encouraging transparency including what is done to what effect in field work agencies in which students are placed and ensuring that students acquire critical appraisal skills, assertion skills to use them and feedback needed to enhance expertise (Rousmaniere, Goodyear, Miller, & Wampold 2017). Far more attention should be given to the close link between evidentiary and ethical issues – to the ethics of risk, drawing on relevant research (e.g. about the importance of feedback) and discussions of moral reasoning in other professions (e.g. Chambers 2011; Ståhl, Zaal, & Skitka 2016). A course should be required on "Avoidable ignorance in social work".

Involve clients as informed participants in shared decision-making

It is the service provider's responsibility to involve clients as informed participants including risks of assessment and diagnostic procedures such as false positives. Related information should be available in waiting rooms (e.g. on computers, in brochures and on user-friendly agency websites). Each agency's website should clearly describe the evidentiary status of services used. For any service provider, we should examine the gaps between the services they provide and what should be provided based on related research findings and acceptability of services to clients. We should examine the websites of each agency to identify gaps in information needed to enable informed decision-making and what is provided. Are decision aids available? Are clients informed about the track record of staff to whom they are referred in achieving hoped-for outcomes? All sources should be examined regarding the quality of information provided (e.g. completeness, accuracy, clarity, readability and availability in multiple languages). Increased client involvement may reveal that outcomes of concern to clients are not addressed. This may reveal inequities such as lack of access to lawyers (Wexler 2016). Yet another way to involve clients is to establish accessible, accountable, timely, complaint systems.

Blow the whistle on ethical violations

What do parents and children risk when they come to the attention of a child welfare agency? Should each child welfare office display potential risks on their websites such as the risk that social workers will not accurately understand client strengths, challenges and problems and will not accurately inform clients about the evidentiary status of services used? Only by exposing avoidable harms to children and families is apathy likely to be challenged. Countless reports are written and hundreds of books and articles appear in the professional literature. Yet clear avoidable ignorance that contributes to risk to children and families is neglected. Other routes must be pursued such as working together with client advocates to expose ethical lapses and related daily injustices and pressing for meaningful accountability requirements in legislation. Each agency should urge staff to bring harmful or ineffective services to others' attention, including related fraud and corruption. Many avoidable risks in child welfare call for "outrage" which can be an important motivating factor in whistleblowing (e. g, Malisow 2016). Goal displacement, such as making money at the expense of helping clients (institutional corruption), is more likely to continue if not revealed by blowing the whistle on harmful policies and practices. This will be easier in some contexts compared with others (e.g. Skivenes & Trygstad 2010). Each agency should establish clear policies that reward rather than punish whistleblowers (Ash 2016). Advocacy organisations such as Childrens' Rights can be involved to file lawsuits to seek reform. (See www.childrensrights.org.) Parents' rights groups can be involved (Franklin 2016).

In conclusion

The ethics of risk requires us to recognise how avoidable ignorance may contribute to avoidable risks to children and families and take steps to minimise it, taking advantage of critical thinking values, knowledge and skills including the vital role of criticism. It requires us to identify and learn from our mistakes and to decide together with others, how related ethical dilemmas can best be handled including critically appraising the morality of excuses offered for not acting to minimise avoidable risk. Currently, there is silence about the many ways in which avoidable ignorance contributes to avoidable risk to children and families including ignoring known knowns (ineffective practices) as well as known unknowns (competence of staff). There is a continuing reluctance to be transparent regarding what is done to what effect including failure to honour informed consent obligations. The plethora of published material may contribute to an illusion that avoidable harms are being revealed and addressed when they are not. Revealing avoidable ignorance would be economically and politically unpopular to many involved parties. This points to the importance of creating organisational and educational cultures as well as effective governmental accountability measures that encourage systemic attention to decreasing harmful avoidable ignorance.

It has been said: "Where there is a will, there is a way". I suggest that we know a great deal about "the way" – to reveal and minimise avoidable ignorance that contributes to avoidable risk to children and families, guided by our ethical obligations. Informed consent requires being informed ourselves – about ignorance as well as knowledge and sharing important uncertainties with clients. We can bring avoidable ignorance that contributes to avoidable risks to the attention of all involved parties; that is, increase transparency of what is done to what effect as required by ethical obligations. We can (and should) involve clients as informed participants. We can discontinue funding of programmes of unknown effectiveness and those that harm clients and use the money saved to offer services that have been critically tested and found to decrease risk to children and families (Prasad & Ioannidis 2014). We can provide education and tools needed to act ethically. We can arrange governmental accountability policies and organisational cultures and climates that encourage staff to act ethically. We can provide services that we ourselves would welcome.

References

Allen, K. (2015, April 17). Reducing inappropriate psychotropic prescribing for children and youth in foster care. *Health Affairs Blog*, pp. 1–4.

Angel, M. (2011, June 23). The epidemic of mental illness: Why? *New York Review of Books*.

Ash, A. (2016). *Whistleblowing and ethics in health and social care*. London: Jessica Kingsley.

Barth, R. P., Landsverk, J., Chamberlain, P., Reid, J. B., Rolls, J. A., Hurlburt, M. S., ... Kohl, P. L. (2005). Parent-training programs in child welfare services: Planning for a more evidence-based approach to serving biological parents. *Research on Social Work Practice, 15*, 353–371.

Bartholet, E. (1999). *Nobody's children: Abuse and neglect, foster drift, and the adoption alternative*. Boson: Beacon Press.

Chalmers, I. (2004). Well informed uncertainties about the effects of treatments. *BMJ, 328*, 475–476.

Chambers, D. W. (2011). Developing a self-scoring comprehensive instrument to measure rest's four component model of moral behavior: The Moral Skills Inventory. *Journal of Dental Education, 75*, 23–35.

Cosgrove, L., Bursztajn, H. J., Erlich, D. R., Wheeler, E. E., & Shaughnessy, A. F. (2013). Conflicts of interest and the quality of recommendations in clinical guidelines. *Journal of Evaluation in Clinical Practice, 19*, 674–681.

Dunning, D., Heath, C., & Suls, J. M. (2004). Flawed self-assessment: Implications for health, education, and the work place. *Psychological Science and the Public Interest, 5*, 69–106.

Elwyn, G., Edwards, A., & Thompson, R. (Eds.). (2016). *Shared decision making in health care: Achieving evidence-based patient choice* (3rd ed.). New York, NY: Oxford University Press.

Entwistle, V. A., Sheldon, T. A., Sowden, A., & Watt, I. S. (1998). Evidence-informed patient choice: Practical issues of involving patients in decisions about health care technologies. *International Journal of Technology Assessment in Health Care, 14*, 212–225.

Ericsson, K. A. (2015). Acquisition and maintenance of medical expertise: A perspective from the expert-performance approach with deliberate practice. *Academic Medicine, 90*, 1471–1486.

Franklin, R. (2016). New York child protection courts: Absurd levels of dysfunction. National Parents Organization. Retrieved from 3/4/2017.

Gambrill, E. (2012a). *Propaganda in the helping professions.* New York, NY: Oxford University Press.

Gambrill, E. (2012b). *Critical thinking in clinical practice: Improving the quality of judgments and decisions.* New York, NY: John Wiley & Sons.

Gambrill, E., & Gibbs, L. (2017). *Critical thinking for helping professionals: A skills based workbook* (4th ed.). New York, NY: Oxford University Press.

Gambrill, E., & Shlonsky, A. (2000). Risk assessment in context. *Children and Youth Services Review, 22*(11/12), 813–837.

Gambrill, E., & Shlonsky, A. (2001). The need for comprehensive risk management systems in child welfare. *Children and Youth Services Review, 23*(1), 79–107.

Gigerenzer, G. (2014). *Risk savvy: How to make good decisions.* New York, NY: Viking.

Gigerenzer, G., & Gray, J. A. M. (Ed.). (2011). Launching the century of the patient. In *Better doctors, better patients, better decisions: Envisioning health Care 2020* (pp. 3–28). Cambridge, MA: MIT Press.

Gorman, D. M. (2017). Has the National Registry of Evidence-based Programs and Practices (NREPP) lost its way? *International Journal of Drug Policy, 45*, 40–41.

Ioannidis, J. P. A. (2005). Why most published research findings are false. *PLoS Med, 2*(8), e124.

Ioannidis, J. P. A. (2016). The mass production of redundant, misleading, and conflicted systematic reviews and meta-analyses. *The Milbank Quarterly, 94*, 485–514.

Kempner, J. (2015). The production of forbidden knowledge. In M. Gross & L. McGoey (Eds.), *Routledge international handbook of ignorance studies* (pp. 77–83). New York, NY: Routledge.

Klein, G. (2015). A naturalistic decision making perspective in studying intuitive decision making. *Journal of Applied Research in Memory and Cognition, 4*, 164–168.

Lambert, M. J. (2010). *Prevention of treatment failure: The use of measuring, monitoring, and feedback in clinical practice.* Washington, DC: American Psychological Association.

Lessig, L. (2013). 'Institutional corruption' defined. *The Journal of Law, Medicine & Ethics, 41*, 553–555.

Malisow, C. (2016, February 16). *There's little outrage for 12,000 kids suffering in the Texas foster care system.* Houston Press. Retrieved March 14, 2017.

McGoey, L. (2007). On the will to ignorance in bureaucracy. *Economy and Society, 36*, 212–235.

McGoey, L. (2012). The logic of strategic ignorance. *The British Journal of Sociology, 63*, 553–576.

Miller, S. D., Hubble, M. A., Chow, D., & Seidel, J. (2015). Beyond measures and monitoring: Realizing the potential of feedback-informed treatment. *Psychotherapy, 52*, 449–457.

Munz, P. (1985). *Our knowledge of the growth of knowledge: Popper or Wittgenstein?*. London: Routledge & Kegan Paul.

National Association of Social Workers (2008). *Code of ethics*. Silver Spring, MD: NASW.

New Jersey Office of the Child Advocate. (2008). *Protecting children. A review of investigations of institutional child abuse and neglect*. Trenton, NJ: New Jersey Office of the Public Advocate. Promoting Positive Change for Children.

Obradovic, Z. (2011). *Report on the KIDS system: Review and analysis*.

Perrenoud, B., Velonaki, V. S., Bodenmann, P., & Ramelet, A. S. (2015). The effectiveness of health literacy interventions on the informed consent process of health care users: A systematic review protocol. *JBI Database of Systematic Reviews and Implementation Reports, 10*, 82–94.

Pollack, D., & Popham, G. L. (2009). 'Wrongful death' of children in foster care. *University of La Verne Law Review, 31*(1), 25–44.

Prasad, V., & Ioannidis, J. P. A. (2014). Evidence-based de-implementation for contradicted, unproven, and aspiring healthcare practices. *Implementation Science, 9*, 556.

Purchase of Service Directory. (2014). Honolulu, HI: Department of Human Services Social Services Division.

Rapley, M., Moncrieff, J., & Dillon, J. (Eds.). (2011). *De-medicalizing misery: Psychiatry, psychology and the human condition*. New York, NY: Palgrave Macmillan.

Roston, A. (2015, April 17). Culture of incompetence: For-profit foster-care giant is leaving Illinois. *BuzzFeed*. Retrieved 2/6/17, from www.buzzfeed.com

Roston, A., & Singer-Vine, J. (2015). Fostering profits: A BuzzFeed News investigation identified deaths, sex abuse, and blunders in screening, training, and overseeing foster parents at the nation's largest for-profit foster care company. Retrieved 7/17/17, from www.buzzfeed.com

Rousmaniere, T., Goodyear, R. K., Miller, S. D., & Wampold, B. E. (Eds.). (2017). *Using deliberate practice to improve supervision and training*. Hoboken, NJ: Wiley/Blackwell.

Sackett, D. L., Richardson, W. S., Rosenberg, W., & Haynes, R. B. (1997). *Evidence-based medicine: How to practice and teach EBM*. New York, NY: Churchill Livingstone.

Schwarz, A. (2016). *ADHD Nation: Children, doctors, big pharma, and the making of an American epidemic*. New York, NY: Scribner.

Sheehan, J., & Sherman, K. A. (2012). Computerized decision aids: A systematic review of their effectiveness in facilitating high-quality decision-making in various health-related contexts. *Patient Education and Counseling, 88*, 69–86.

Skivenes, M., & Trygstad, S. C. (2010). When whistle-blowing works: The Norwegian case. *Human Relations, 63*, 1071–1097.

Slovic, P. (Ed.). (2010). *The feeling of risk: New perspectives on risk perception*. New York, NY: Earthscan.

Spratt, T., Devaney, J., & Hayes, D. (2015). In and out of home care decisions: The influence of confirmation bias in developing decision supportive reasoning. *Child Abuse & Neglect, 49*, 76–85.

Ståhl, T., Zaal, M. P., & Skitka, L. J. (2016). Moralized rationality: Relying on logic and evidence in the formation and evaluation of belief can be seen as a moral issue. *PLoS ONE, 11*, e0166332.

Stoesz, D., Karger, H. J., & Carrilio, T. (2010). *A dream deferred: How social work education lost its way and what can be done*. New Brunswick, NJ: Transaction.

Szasz, T. S. (1994). *Cruel compassion: Psychiatric control of society's unwanted*. New York, NY: John Wiley.

Taylor, B. J. (2013). *Professional decision making and risk in social work* (2nd ed.). Los Angeles, CA: Sage.

Thyer, B. A. (2005). The misfortunes of behavioral social work: Misprized, misread, and misconstrued. In. S. A. Kirk (Ed.), *Mental health in the social environment: Critical perspectives* (pp. 330-343). New York: Columbia University Press.

Vincent, C. (2010). The essentials of patient safety (2nd ed.). Wiley-Blackwell – BMJ Books.

Walton, D. (2015). *Goal-based reasoning for argumentation*. New York, NY: Cambridge University Press.

Wampold, B. E., & Imel, Z. E. (2015). *The great psychotherapy debate: The evidence for what makes psychotherapy work* (2nd ed.). New York, NY: Routledge.

Wexler, R. (2016, October 18). Lessons for child welfare from the California 'right-to-lie' case. *The chronicle of social change*, pp. 1–7.

Wulczyn, F., Daro, D., Fluke, J., Feldman, S., Glodek, C., & Lifanda, K. (2010). *Adapting a systems approach to child protection: Key concepts and considerations. Working paper*. New York: United Nations Children's Fund (UNICEF).

Zerubavel, E. (2006). *The elephant in the room: Silence and denial in everyday life*. New York, NY: Oxford University Press.

Mark Hardy

IN DEFENCE OF ACTUARIALISM: INTERROGATING THE LOGIC OF RISK IN SOCIAL WORK PRACTICE

This article presents findings from a study of risk-based decision-making which challenges aspects of the well-established consensus regarding the role that actuarially generated knowledge plays in risk-based decision-making in social work. Firstly, it suggests that there is little direct relationship between the process of risk assessment and its outcome. Secondly, it highlights that subjective practitioner judgement plays a role in elevating risk levels beyond those which actuarial calculations warrant. Finally, although risk aversion is evident, this cannot be reductively attributed to actuarial knowledge generation strategies. Instead, it is a function of practice in an environment in which fear of blame is a very real concern. I conclude with discussion of the implications of these findings for ongoing debates regarding forms of knowledge in practice.

Introduction

Risk has been an overt concern in social work for approaching 30 years and arguably represents a significant departure from familiar social work concerns. An emphasis on risk pushes social work away from inclusive, emancipatory approaches towards exclusionary, controlling practices which do not necessarily cohere with traditional values. Social work has been transformed from a profession with a commitment to enhancing individual well-being to one concerned to prevent harm, either to service users themselves, or to other members of the community. Although there are various explanations for such shifts, it is arguably no co-incidence that they followed, in the UK at least, the election of a reforming Conservative government in the late 1970's, determined to establish neoliberal principles and practices within the structures and institutions of government, with a corresponding impact on 'social' thinking and practices For many, this is a regressive shift, with largely detrimental effects.

In this article, I will report findings from a study of the impact of risk thinking in social work. Although to some extent, this tally with aspects of the dominant narrative regarding the generalised impact of risk thinking on social work practice, they differ quite significantly with regard to the specific role that actuarial knowledge plays in this. Firstly, the data suggests that actually, practitioners elevate risk levels beyond those which actuarial calculations warrant. Relatedly, it highlights that subjective practitioner judgement sometimes drives disempowering judgements, rather than actuarial knowledge. Finally, the data suggests that although risk aversion is, indeed, evident, this cannot be reductively attributed to actuarial knowledge generation strategies. Whatever social work's 'ill's', it seems that these are distinct from the role played by actuarial knowledge, which sometimes represents a potentially valuable source of knowledge for practice, and a counterweight against risk aversion.

Background

Various scholars have outlined the changes to social work associated with the rise of neoliberal thinking across the institutions and practices of government. Webb (2006), emphasised how the logics of risk, regulation and security intersect with neoliberal perspectives regarding choice, autonomy and individual responsibility. These differ markedly from the collectivist commitments that inform social work, and so their rise to prominence has impacted in ways which arguably compromise its integrity. Risk, it is argued, accentuates social exclusion, prompts over reliance on coercive approaches to practice, downgrades the significance of social context, and undermines longstanding commitments to social justice (Parton & Kirk 2010). Because of its predominant focus on potential harmful events the energies and resources of practitioners are future-oriented, to the detriment of the here and now. Risk also privileges organisational legitimacy ahead of the right, proper or moral response to individuals facing difficult circumstances. The nature of the services offered by social work agencies emphasise emphasising the rights of the wider community ahead of service user rights. The significance of social context is replaced by a concern with pre-harm (Zedner 2006) and 'prepression', whereby risk 'archives' form the knowledge base for categorisation for pre-emptive intervention (Schinkel 2011). Judgements are informed by cumulative banks of data drawn from similarly categorised populations rather than the particular details of a case as interpreted by the professional. Significantly, as a result, social work has become risk averse. Practitioners become participants in a repressive framework, 'unreflective co-conspirators' in the politics of risk. The logic of risk functions as a 'predominantly morally conservative and repressive social, political and cultural force in contemporary social work' (Stanford 2008, p.209).

Risk in social work practice

Although the notion of 'risk' originally referred to the probability of any particular event occurring, in social work it has come to refer to the likelihood of a negative outcome – such as a child death, a suicide, harm to a vulnerable adult or the commission of violence by a service user. Social workers are now required to assess the likelihood of such outcomes occurring in particular cases, and take appropriate action to prevent their occurrence. How they might best do this remains contentious.

The trajectory which the development of approaches to risk assessment has followed in social work practice is similar to that in other domains, albeit with its own distinctive features. First generation approaches are sometimes referred to as clinical approaches, wherein a practitioner makes a judgement as to whether or not a particular service user poses a risk to themselves or others on the basis of their understanding of that person and their situation gleaned from the relationship they have established, case records and ongoing interpersonal contact. These approaches have their roots in holistic, needs based approaches to assessment, whereby 'practitioners ... relied almost entirely on intuition, experience and individual judgement to make their risk-based decisions' (Turner & Colombo 2008, p.166). However, unstructured clinical judgement came to be problematised, due to concerns that professional discretion masked biased judgements (Monahan 1981) and so more effective risk assessment processes and tools were sought.

Second generation actuarial approaches to risk assessment are very different. They utilise statistical analysis of relationships between social and psychological variables to calculate probabilities at population level. Practitioners input data regarding static and dynamic variables, history and context, into a software programme which results in a percentage score – the likelihood of harm – or banding – low, medium, high or similar configuration. Such knowledge has been characterised as 'an anchor against the force of bias' (Jones & Plowman 2005, p.135). Quinsey, Harris, Rice, and Cormier provocatively suggest 'the complete replacement of existing practice with actuarial methods' (1998, p.22) with practitioners deliberately disengaged so as to establish objective, reliable and scientific assessments.

A major limitation of second generation tools, however, is that their results lack specificity when applied to a person or family rather than to a population, raising questions about the extent they are useful in working with individuals. Nor do they provide indicators regarding intervention or risk management because they are not based upon dynamic associations. There is also a suggestion that they encourage an inflated sense of expertise among practitioners, given that 'the pseudo-scientific nature of this process is undoubtedly seductive' (Turner & Colombo 2008, p.169). In mainstream social work, then 'structured clinical judgement' is now often the preferred approach in some settings, combining research-based considerations, including actuarial knowledge, with knowledge of the individual service user that the practitioner has by virtue of clinical experience. These third generation approaches integrate clinical and actuarial information, on the basis that the advantages of each potentially outweigh their respective limitations.

In theory, then, first generation approaches to risk assessment rely solely on clinical, subjective judgement. Second generation approaches entail the straightforward application of actuarial scoring based on objective knowledge. Third generation tools seek to ensure that the strengths and limitations of clinical and actuarial approaches more adequately counter balance each other by drawing on both objective and subjective knowledge. In reality these approaches have been used variably depending on the context in which practitioners are required to undertake risk assessments. Arguably, in UK settings, clinical and structured approaches remain generally dominant, although, in some contexts, there are initiatives which seek to formalise and objectify the process and outcomes of assessment. The insistence that actuarial scoring be incorporated tends to be limited to work with known offenders – domestic violence, forensic mental health, dual diagnosis, etc. Youth justice and probation practitioners, for example, utilise 'hybrid' needs/risk approaches to assessment (Case & Haines 2009, Deering 2011).

Explaining risk

How and why have such changes come about and with what consequences? There are notable theoretical attempts to address these questions. Generally, these have a macro level emphasis and emphasise the impact of social, cultural and technological change on society. Certain authors have become synonomous with discussion of risk, and I will not rehearse the positions of Beck, Giddens, Douglas, etc., here. Suffice to say that such authors agree that, paradoxically, modernity provokes 'new' hazards and changes perceptions of risk and in the process undermines societal faith in the expertise of science and the professions. In seeking to understand the impact of risk on social practices such as social work, however, it is important to critically interrogate the links between changing political priorities and policy and practice (Marston & Macdonald 2006). Here, I will draw on some of the more influential theoretical perspectives which seek to explain the significance of these developments for social work.

The death of the social

A relationship between social transformations and policy and practice is suggested in Nikolas Rose's influential analysis (1996). Here, the logics of social government are problematised and reformulated. The changing nature of social provision reflects a decline in faith in the skills and knowledge of social professionals. This results from the confluence of ideology and a lack of empirical evidence of effectiveness. The solution to 'the problem of welfare' entails a shift from 'social' to 'economic' reasoning, choice and individual responsibility. Under advanced liberalism, capable and responsible citizens will prudentially secure against risk. Practitioners assume responsibility for applying risk criteria to differentiate 'the prudent from the imprudent self, the self able to manage itself from the self who must be managed by others' (Rose 1996, p.14) via 'dividing practices', including risk assessment. Prediction replaces diagnosis, and practitioners are reconstituted as 'control agents' with an explicit role 'to minimise the riskiness of the most risky' (Rose 1999, p.260).

Despite a relative lack of faith in clinical effectiveness, there is nevertheless a belief that security can be furthered via administrative methods. The 'power of the single figure' (Rose 1998, p.187) assumes key significance and so traditional associations with 'artful', subjective practice are replaced by claims to knowledge which attest to their own objectivity. Rather than 'care or cure', practitioners encourage self-management (Howe 2009). The role of the practitioner becomes primarily an informational one:

> As the logic of prediction comes to replace the logic of diagnosis … professionals become, in certain fundamental senses, knowledge workers, engaged in the accumulation, calibration, classification and interpretation and communication of information relevant to judgements about risk (Rose 1998, p.185).

From dangerousness to risk

Historically, dangerousness has been assessed categorically and clinically – an individual either is or is not dangerous, and that judgement is best made by an appropriately qualified practitioner (Castel 1991). However, this distinction came to be seen as problematic, especially as 'care in the community' accelerated across the domains of social work, provoking anxieties about behaviour, capacity and functioning post-deinstitutionalisation. Actuarialism offered a solution, by rendering the knowledge claims of professionals probabilistic rather than absolute. Thus risk thinking 'dissolve[s] the notion of a subject or a concrete individual, and put in its place a combinatory of *factors*, the factors of risk' such that 'the essential component of intervention no longer takes the form of the direct face-to-face relationship between the … professional and the client' but instead concerns 'flows of population based on the collation of a range of abstract factors deemed liable to produce risk' (Castel 1991, p.281). Relatedly, information supplants expertise as essential to the fulfilment of agency objectives. The traditional skills and knowledge of the practitioner are downplayed by a shift 'from the gaze to the objective accumulation of facts' (Castel 1991, p.282) as practice is reconstituted as 'a *new mode of surveillance*: that of systematic predetection' (ibid, p.288). The relationship between practitioner and subject is less important because the subject has been supplanted and reconstructed from risk factors. Their detection can be imputed from statistical correlations. The presence of risk is indicative of a need for intervention, but the nature of this also shifts from the transformational to the managerial, and entails the use of 'technologies' that enable processes of categorisation as a basis for differentiation in the service of prevention and security.

Consequently, it is argued that there has been an explicit assimilation of social work into wider 'regimes of control'. Actuarialism represents a 'managerial attempt to regulate … the overall probability of undesirable conduct' (Rose 2002, p.9). Castel suggests that these 'preventative strategies of social administration … depart in a profoundly innovatory way from the traditions of … social work' (1991, p.281).

From the social to the informational

There is a parallel strand of theorising which explores the role of technology in accelerating the shift towards risk. Franko Aas (2005a) analysed the ways in which developments in I.T. impacted on sentencing practice. Subsequently, this remit has expanded to examine the role, content and function of changing forms of knowledge within decision-making across domains and jurisdictions. Parton (2008) suggests that such rapid developments have impacted significantly on the nature and form of knowledge drawn upon. Reliance on formal rather than informal knowledge sources means that social work decision-making is positioned as an objective process based upon factual knowledge. Risk becomes an 'artefact' phenomena which 'exist [s] in the formulae, theorems or assessments which construct them' (Parton 1996, p.111).

Webb suggests that 'Actuarialism refers to the suite or programme of risk calculation techniques that underpin social interventions in advanced liberal societies' (2009, p.210). Certain presumptions underpin faith in the basis for and accuracy of calculation: firstly, that it is possible to predict *future* behaviour of individuals on the basis of *past* behaviour of populations, using statistical aggregates of 'risk factors'; next, these judgements are more likely to be accurate when based on *objective* rather than *subjective* knowledge – numbers 'act as technical mechanisms for making judgments' (Rose

1999, p.198); finally, outcomes will be improved if decision-making draws on *actuarial* rather than *clinical* sources, based on formal rather than informal knowledge. Consequently, data and information are privileged ahead of relational understanding such that 'complex explanatory narratives tend to be compressed into shorter, instantly understandable messages' (Franko Aas 2005b, p.152). Holism becomes redundant as 'master categories ... obscure any ambiguities' (Parton & Kirk 2010, p.33). Consequently, practitioners 'have no overall perspective relating to the total life situation and biography of the client' (Fitzgibbon 2007, p.88). With the emergence of actuarialism in social work, 'individuals are reduced to end oriented practices that are configured by a form of political arithmetic' (Webb 2009, p.223). The logic of risk, then, plays a key role in a shift from inclusion to exclusion, from care to control.

The study

The findings in this article derive from a qualitative study which investigated if, how and why concerns about risk have impacted on the theory and practice of work within various domains of social work. The fieldwork – completed in 2011 – addressed the relative paucity of research into risk *from the perspective of the social work practitioner* (Barry 2007). It entailed two inter-related strands. Firstly, detailed genealogical case studies, which, following Foucault (1977), analyse the origins and development of theory and practice in mental health social work, forensic social work and probation practice as a basis for constructing a 'history of the present'. Secondly, in-depth qualitative interviews with 29 practitioners, from three domains of practice, in both community and institutional settings in northern England. Sites were selected according to a theoretical purposive logic, with respondents taken as having knowledge and expertise regarding if and how 'risk thinking' has brought about effects in the operation of power and authority in practice. Key questions that arise include 'what forms of thought, knowledge, expertise ... means of calculation, or rationality are employed in practices of governing?' (Dean 1999, p.31). My focus, then is on the forms and sources of knowledge which practitioners draw upon in making decisions regarding risk. In what ways do these correspond with the 'generation' of tool used in particular agencies, according to the underpinning logic of risk? And how do practitioners perceive this as affecting the processes and outcomes of risk-based decision-making? I will structure the presentation of data around certain themes. Firstly, the role that the logic of risk – as manifest in the risk 'technology' used in each domain – plays in the process of risk-based decision-making. Secondly, the extent to which risk aversion is evident in practice and how this intersects with the forms of knowledge underpinning risk-based decision-making; and thirdly, the extent to which in this study risk aversion appears to be a function of subjective rather than objective knowledge. Although space precludes full exposition, in what follows I have nevertheless sought to do justice to the preponderance of perspectives within the data.

The logic of risk in practice

The 'logic of risk' suggests that levels of practitioner discretion in determining risk status in a particular case vary according to the variety of 'tool' utilised in a particular context, here conceived of as a continuum from pure clinical judgement to unassailed actuarial science. The data suggests that matters are more complicated than this. Although there certainly were instances of practitioners using assessment tools in ways which corresponded with stated intentions, what was most notable was the extent to which practitioner accounts problematised the assumption that the generation of tool influenced in any deterministic way the decisions that practitioners make.

Clinical judgement (Forensic mental health)

Here, it was clear that practitioners did not necessarily determine the risk status on the basis of subjective knowledge alone. Instead, they described numerous systems and practices which impacted upon the operation of clinical judgement in its pure form. For example, they drew upon formalised actuarial assessments undertaken by other disciplines in their own judgements.

> We do our own clinical assessment based on what we know about the patients, but we do draw on what the psychologists have had to say too, and the nurses. They use VRAG and SORAG or Hare on the personality disorder ward so we take that into account too, they have a different perspective (Forensic social worker (FSW)).

Individual assessment was supplemented by high levels of reliance on case discussions with peers, team managers and other professionals cross referencing their own views with the opinions of others, as well as risk assessment tools developed specifically for violent service users in criminal and forensic settings.

> It's quite a responsibility when you think about it, not the sort of thing to work out on your own, and why would you anyway, there's a lot of people involved (FSW).

Practitioners routinely referred to case discussions in team meetings and in supervision, as well as multi-disciplinary and multi-agency fora, including MAPPA, and the effects inter-professional discussion had in informing both individual and collective determination of risk status.

Actuarial tools (Mental health social work)

Here, there was an evident mismatch between the dominant narrative and how actuarial scores are actually utilised within decision-making. Practitioners did acknowledge that actuarial knowledge had certain advantages.

> Decisions … need to be accurate and backed up and so tools can be helpful. I wouldn't feel comfortable just guessing (Mental health social worker (MHSW)).

Here, clinical judgement is equated with guesswork, which is – by implication – inferior to other approaches, and so there is an ethical imperative to ensure that decision-making is informed by more rigorous forms of knowledge. This is also the case below.

> The tool … gets you to structure what you know and what you think is backed up.
> It's important that we use them cos our decisions make a real difference for people
> so we can't afford to miss things or just make assumptions (MHSW).

Despite recognition of the possible value of actuarial knowledge, and although
practitioners did undertake scoring, this was not routinely used as a basis for determining risk status. Although the agency represented itself as utilising second generation approaches, there was no actual requirement that actuarial scoring be applied
deterministically in judgements of risk status. Instead, actuarial scores informed clinical
judgement, rather than ruled it. For example:

> There's a policy, but its not, you know, the law, and that's probably right, cos its
> helpful but not 'the truth' or infallible, sometimes it doesn't apply to that particular
> person (MHSW).

The issue here is specificity, an acknowledged limitation of the sort of population
level knowledge that actuarial scoring generates.

> I do it, and I know that's supposed to be it, that's the point of piloting it, but its not
> the custom and sometimes its so obviously not right that yes we take it into account
> but because its not specific to that person, then who knows, you've still got to make
> your own mind up (MHSW).

Thus, even where an agency had explicitly decided to use a tool which in theory
should limit the role of subjective knowledge, in practice this is still allowed for.

Needs / risk hybrid (Probation service)

Although third generation approaches arguably enable the tensions between informal
and formal knowledge sources to be balanced (Robinson 2003), it was evident that
individual practitioners' perceptions of their utility varied considerably. It was notable
that the presumed ability of such tools to balance competing variables led to 'new'
practice dilemmas, especially regarding the weighting of actuarial knowledge derived
from static variables and clinical assessments of the mediating or escalating effects of
dynamic factors. Practitioners interpreted these weightings in varied fashion. Although
this corresponds with the logic underpinning this approach, this manifested in ways
which were probably unforeseen:

> It's tricky because you know it's supposed to be robust but you get different views
> depending on whether someone gets on with him, when, obviously, well its not
> consistent, is it. But that's what happens (Probation officer (PO)).

One of the factors which might determine an offender's risk status, it appears, is
whether or not a practitioner likes that individual at a personal level.

Other practitioners found the expectation that they integrate their own subjective
views with actuarial knowledge frustrating or frightening. Some were concerned at the
possible consequences of suggesting that actuarial estimates were too high.

If you've got an actual score that says there's like, a seventy per cent likelihood of reoffending it's really hard to justify saying, well, despite that he'll be alright, cos that could come back to haunt you, why did you over rule the score? (PO).

Significantly, although other practitioners sometimes welcomed the opportunity that inclusion of subjective judgement allows, they were hesitant in doing so:

You do need to be careful if you're downgrading the risk status, you're taking a risk doing it (PO).

This accords with Witkin's (2017) belief that risk is a risk for social work practitioners.

In this setting, then both clinical and actuarial knowledge inform decision-making, but it is clear that these influences do not function deterministically. The integration of different forms of knowledge depends on factors that the individual practitioner chooses to privilege.

Risk aversion

Perhaps more than any other factor, it is concern about risk aversion which underpins many of the concerns that critics have expressed regarding the role of actuarial knowledge in social work practice (Fitzgibbon 2011). Actuarialism quantifies risk, with numeric values 'purporting to act as technical mechanisms for making judgements' (Rose 1999, p.198). This makes them more difficult to disregard. In settings in which the logic of risk is predominant and practitioner discretion constrained via reliance on actuarial scoring, practitioners are more likely to err on the side of the caution, over-estimate risk and avoid positive risk taking (Peay 2003). Although practitioners spoke of the dilemmas involved in risk-based decision-making, and of the strategies they adopted to limit the impact of concerns about risk on their decision-making, even so, risk averse practice is common.

This is not to suggest that all social workers are always risk averse. Practitioners also described situations in which they did seek to practice 'positive risk taking'.

I'm supposed to be on the lookout for signs of non-compliance, florid symptoms, deterioration. But if I did something every time there was a 'blip', there'd be no point letting them out in the first place. They're constantly testing you, but they have to if they're going to adapt back to living in the community. Otherwise they're over dependent and can't function (MHSW).

Elsewhere, practitioners suggested that there is still a concern with issues of fairness in decision-making, which would not be the case if the precautionary principle was wholly dominant.

We always weigh up the positives and negatives. If you just looked at what might go wrong you'd never do anything for anyone. I've had a few times when it's clearly been unfair, cos we're worried for ourselves really, but most of the time it's fine (FSW).

Nevertheless, the ability of practitioners to resist risk averse tendencies was constrained. Top down concerns filter down to practitioner level.

> It's not that I'm against taking risks, you have to judge how to proceed. But the context is definitely very harsh and you can't ignore people's worries. We've certainly tightened up, stuff that was custom and practice is rare now (FSW).

Feelings of vulnerability are thus countered by adhering to policy. Similar concerns are apparent in probation work.

> If someone is going to hurt someone, I need to do something now. Usually, that means getting them back in. It's better to be safe than sorry, I know it's a cliché but it is (PO).

Similarly, mental health social workers referred to instances in which criteria for access were applied tightly because of concerns regarding the possible risk posed by patients being discharged.

> Sometimes they just won't wait, and you can be in trouble. Ideally, everything should be in place before they come out and we're sometimes able to delay it, cos if something goes wrong and it comes out we just let it go ahead without stuff in place we'll be properly liable (MHSW).

There were also suggestions that there was a justifiable need for practice to become more risk averse, given previous service failures. This entailed shifts in positioning in the enduring debate regarding 'care vs. control' (Howe 2015).

> It's always a difficult balance, but we need to learn from mistakes and that probably does mean not taking as many chances, not being quite so optimistic. That does mean … clients will pay a price but maybe that's as it should be (MHSW).

> Therapeutic optimism is all well and good but you've got to realise most people do relapse, we know that, we can't pretend they don't and we need to take that into account (FSW).

Fear of false negatives

It was also apparent that potential false positives – intervening to address a potential risk that does not materialise – do not concern practitioners in the way that false negatives – not intervening to prevent harm – do. Media, political and managerial scrutiny focuses on false negatives as exemplifying 'service failure'. In the main, this seemed to be because there is no way of demonstrating that a false positive has actually occurred.

> You might make the wrong decision, but you wouldn't know. Either you're right and cos they're 'in' nothing happens, or you're wrong but they're still in and nothing happens. You can't know, so it's pretty academic really (FSW).

Similarly,

> We're bound to be wrong sometimes, but there's no way of knowing, it's not like you can do an experiment to work it out. I suppose that's where tribunals come in, to make sure you're not being too cautious. But day-to-day it's not something my managers hassling me about (MHSW).

The suggestion here is that as there is no practical means of establishing whether or not a judgement made by a practitioner has led to a false positive, this does not intrude into decision-making to anything like the extent that corresponding concerns regarding the possibility of false negatives might. This conundrum is summed up by Castel: 'When in doubt it is better to act, since, even if unfounded intervention is an error, it is one that will certainly never be known as such' (1991, p. 283).

Fear of blame

Thus the logic of actuarialism is not the principal influence on tendencies towards risk aversion evident in the data. This pointed instead to the role played by practitioners' own concerns regarding the potential consequences for themselves should a false negative occur – or fear of blame.

Various practitioners pointed to the role that a hostile media plays in contributing to a climate of fear for practitioners.

> You see in Community Care … naming and shaming incompetent workers. And there's the press and the news too, they're always hard line. It's a real worry because obviously mistakes are inevitable and have real effects, and for us too (PO).

> Being on the front page of the Daily Mail, journalists on the doorstep, my kids being hassled. I know it's unlikely but that's the fear, they blame individual workers. And I'm not confident that management would protect me … there's a real sense that its 'look after number one'. It's natural, even, you have to put yourself first, and if that has implications for the clients, then so be it (MHSW).

There is a real sense that practitioners regard agency management as sometimes abandoning practitioners to their fate:

> There's been inquiries after serious incidents, they go through your records, it doesn't matter if you've covered the biggies, you've still got to make sure everything's been done by the book cos little minor things that you miss every day look bad when it goes wrong (PO).

This practitioner is suggesting that it is not the quality of practice which determines whether or not blame is attached to a practitioner, but the extent to which policy and procedure have been adhered to. These may have played little or no part in a serious incident, but with hindsight come to assume inflated significance. Other practitioners elaborated on how this fear intrudes at a personal level.

I didn't used to be actually scared. Now if I've been out of the office for more than a few days I'm literally terrified of going in cos I don't know what might have happened. And I'm not lax, but that doesn't mean I can control someone's behaviour, but that's the expectation. And I find myself more concerned about what might happen to me than them, which is the wrong way round (PO).

Despite these misgiving, there was also (somewhat ironic) faith in the power of policy, procedure and protocol to protect practitioners.

That's where policy comes in. If you've stuck to it there'll still be mistakes but you're covered. I'd think most people stick to policy these days. You might not get everything done in time or much cop but when they're high risk they take priority cos if you don't…and if you've stuck to the policy there's no dilemma anyway cos it's pretty straightforward, do things properly and don't take risks (MHSW).

Such a perspective, taken to its logical conclusion, would certainly inhibit scope for positive risk taking.

Here, then, practitioners are testifying to the effects that the context within which they work impacts on the judgements that they make regarding the risk a service user poses. The consequences for service users were clear in how practitioners described how their own subjective interpretation of the intersection between the personal and professional impacted upon their judgements.

It's not as though he actually met the criteria, because on OGRS [actuarial scoring tool] he was quite low and he was certainly low risk of harm. But sometimes you just get a feeling, its worrying … what if … and so I upped him to high risk and eventually he was recalled (PO).

Its your job on the line, you have to be careful. There are people who you just know are risky. The tool might say something else, but you know them, so that's high and that's that (MHSW).

It is sometimes suggested that a return to relational practice, in which clinical judgement is key, might be a remedy for risk aversion and promote positive risk taking. Here, it appears that the opposite is the case. Practitioner suggest quite explicitly that they draw on their own subjective clinical judgement to elevate risk levels beyond those which actuarial scoring suggests is appropriate. It seems then that associations between the logic of risk, in its actuarial form, and risk aversion are not as straightforwardly as is sometimes assumed. Rather, the use of subjective knowledge sometimes enables practice which deviates markedly from the forms of 'subversive' (Fook 2002, p.147) but constructive practice which proponents of 'artful' social work tend to equate with clinical judgement.

Discussion

It is evident then, that in the agencies in which this research was conducted there is no straightforward correlation between the generation of 'technology' used and the actual process followed in risk-based decision-making, which must be accounted for by factors other than 'the logic of risk'. In particular, respondents routinely referred to how their subjective views intersect with concerns regarding their own personal and professional well-being to impact on decisions regarding risk status. It seems fair to conclude that such judgements are, indeed, 'risk averse'. It is also clear, however, that evident risk aversion results from the context within which practitioners are making judgements, which is characterised by a quite pervasive, generalised 'fear of blame'. Parton (1998) identified the influence of 'blaming systems' on social work two decades ago, and it seems that these remain significant. It is also important, I think, that it is not the logic of actuarialism which necessarily promotes risk aversion. The continued significance of subjective practitioner knowledge to risk-based decision-making, particularly in over-ruling actuarially generated knowledge and elevating risk levels, raises doubts about the preferred remedy to risk aversion that many critics of the rise of risk call for. A renaissance in relational practice – whatever its other merits – would do little to promote positive risk taking in a context in which agency concerns regarding the consequences of false negatives mean that fear of blame continue to inform the decision-making of many social workers.

Conclusion

Small scale studies such as this, fixed in time and space, with limited representativeness, generalisability and vulnerable to fluctuations in politics and policy are not well placed to make definitive, wider statements regarding the nature of contemporary practice. They can, however, reasonably raise questions regarding existing, theoretical explanations and perspectives. The findings of this study suggest that existing assumptions regarding the role that actuarially generated knowledge plays in promoting risk aversion in social work may well be misplaced. They also highlight the role that clinical judgement – a sometimes reified notion – can and does play in inhibiting positive risk taking. This should not be too surprising. The original impetus for the use of actuarial method in the social realm stemmed from concerns about injustices associated with untrammelled subjectivity in professional decision-making. This study reminds us of that potential, as well as highlighting the ways in which the context within which practitioners make such decisions can (and does) make the job of social work more difficult than it might otherwise be.

The continued – and possibly escalating – effects of blame culture on practitioner decision-making rest on two misguided assumptions. Firstly, they assume that practitioner decision-making is 'poor' and that blame is therefore deserved when things go wrong, while reform and regulation are required to ensure it does not. In fact, there is little evidence to suggest that social workers are any worse (or better) at assessing risk than any other professional group. Secondly, they intersect with a pervasive but unwarranted expectation of infallibility. The roots of this expectation reflect dominant neoliberal perspectives regarding individuality and responsibility and a clear emphasis within 'new' public management that accountability and value for money within public service practice (as was) requires 'excellence' in all activities. There is little room here for uncertainty, ambiguity or imperfection, and so it is unsurprising that social workers are fearful about the consequences of being seen to make the wrong decision.

Whereas for some, the future of social work ought to be clinical, it is clear that the dichotomous distinction between 'clinical' and 'actuarial', or 'art' and 'science', is not helpful. Knowledge generated 'scientifically' is by no means certain (Firestein 2012). In making the best possible judgement (which is different from a judgement perceived to be accurate) practitioners must integrate knowledge from an array of sources (Evans & Hardy 2010; Pawson, Boaz, Grayson, Long, & Barnes 2003). Actuarial methods represent just one source of knowledge in social work, and as such should not be reified. Debates regarding the relative merits of actuarial and clinical approaches to risk assessment are an example of the truly enduring nomothetic/idiographic tension within the philosophy of knowledge, and we should not expect its exemplification in contemporary social work to resolve this. At best actuarial knowledge provides a base line comparator against which to compare the real people social workers work with: 'the world of pure probability does not exist except on paper … it has nothing to do with breathing, sweating anxious and creative human beings struggling to find their way out of the darkness' (Pratt 2016). We certainly should not over emphasise its rigour or specificity. In fact, actuarial knowledge exposes the limits of science, not least its sometimes limited practical utility (Firestein 2015). It is in the integration of knowledge – actuarial, clinical, formal, informal, subjective and objective – that good social work practice *of necessity* prospers. And as social work pushes at the limits of science, we must also surely continue to acknowledge its debt to the realms of art, philosophy and imagination.

References

Barry, M. (2007). *Effective approaches to risk assessment in social work: An international literature review*. Edinburgh: Scottish Executive.

Case, S., & Haines, K. (2009). *Understanding youth offending: Risk factor research, policy and practice*. Cullompton: Willan.

Castel, R. (1991). From dangerousness to risk. In G. Burchell, C. Gordon, & P. Miller (Eds.), *The Foucault effect: Studies in governmentality* (pp. 281–298). Hemel Hempstead: Harvester Wheatsheaf.

Dean, M. (1999). *Governmentality: Power and rule in modern society*. London: Sage.

Deering, J. (2011). *Probation practice and the new penology*. Farnham: Ashgate.

Evans, T., & Hardy, M. (2010). *Evidence and knowledge for practice*. Cambridge: Polity.

Firestein, S. (2012). *Ignorance: How it drives science*. Oxford: Oxford University Press.

Firestein, S. (2015). *Failure: Why science is so successful*. Oxford: Oxford University Press.

Fitzgibbon, D. W. (2007). Risk analysis and the new practitioner. *Punishment & Society, 9*(1), 87–97.

Fitzgibbon, D. W. (2011). *Probation and social work on trial*. Basingstoke: Palgrave Macmillan.

Fook, J. (2002). *Social work: A critical approach to practice*. London: Sage.

Foucault, M. (1977). *Discipline and punish: The birth of the prison*. London: Allen Lane.

Franko Aas, K. (2005a). *Sentencing in the age of information: From faust to macintosh*. London: The GlassHouse Press.

Franko Aas, K. (2005b). The ad and the form: Punitiveness and technological culture. In J. Pratt, D. Brown, M. Borwn, S. Hallsworth, & W. Morrison (Eds.), *The new punitiveness: Trends, theories, perspectives* (pp. 150–166) Cullompton: Willan.

Howe, D. (2009). *A Brief Introduction to Social Work Theory*. Basingstoke: Palgrave Macmilan.

Howe, D. (2015). *The compleat social worker*. London: Palgrave Macmillan.

Jones, J., & Plowman, C. (2005). Risk assessment: A multidisciplinary approach to estimating harmful behaviour in mentally disordered offenders. In S. Wix & M. Humphreys (Eds.), *Multidisciplinary working in forensic mental health* (pp. 133–150). London: Elsevier.

Marston, G., & Macdonald, C. (2006). Introduction: Reframing social policy analysis. In G. Marston & C. Macdonald (Eds.), *Analysing social policy* (pp. 1–18). Cheltenham: Edward Elgar.

Monahan, J. (1981). *Predicting violent behaviour*. Beverley Hills: Sage.

Parton, N. (1996). Social work, risk and the 'blaming system'. In N. Parton (Ed.), *Social theory, social change and social work* (pp. 98–114). London: Routledge.

Parton, N. (1998). Risk, advanced liberalism and child welfare: The need to rediscover uncertainty and ambiguity. *British Journal of Social Work, 28*, 5–27.

Parton, N. (2008). Changes in the form of knowledge in social work: From the social to the 'informational'? *British journal of social work, 38*, 253–269.

Parton, N., & Kirk, S. (2010). The nature and purposes of social work. In I. Shaw, K. Briar-Lawson, J. Orme, & R. Ruckdeschel (Eds.), *The SAGE handbook of social work research* (pp. 23–36). London: Sage.

Pawson, R., Boaz, A., Grayson, L., Long, A., & Barnes, C. (2003). *Types and quality of knowledge in social care*. London: SCIE.

Peay, J. (2003). *Decisions and dilemmas: Working with mental health law*. Oxford: Hart.

Pratt, J. (2016). Risk control, rights and legitimacy in the limited liability state. *British journal of criminology, 57*(6), 1322–1339.

Quinsey, V. L., Harris, G., Rice, M. E., & Cormier, C. (1998). *Violent offenders: Appraising and managing risk*. Washington, DC: American Psychological Association.

Robinson, G. (2003). Technicality and indeterminacy in probation practice: A case study. *British Journal of Social Work, 35*, 593–610.

Rose, N. (1996). The death of the social? Reconfiguring the territory of government. *Economy and Society, 25*, 327–356.

Rose, N. (1998). Governing risky individuals: The role of psychiatry in new regimes of control. *Psychiatry, Psychology and Law, 5*, 177–195.

Rose, N. (1999). *Powers of freedom: Reframing political thought*. Cambridge: Cambridge University Press.

Rose, N. (2002). Society, madness and control. In A. Buchanan (Ed.), *Care of the mentally disordered offender in the community* (pp. 3–25). Oxford: Oxford University Press.

Schinkel, W. (2011). Pre-pression: The actuarial archive and new technologies of security. *Theoretical Criminology, 15*(4), 365–380.

Stanford, S. (2008). Taking a stand or playing it safe?: Resisting the moral conservatism of risk in social work practice. *European Journal of Social Work, 11*, 209–220.

Turner, T., & Colombo, A. (2008). Risk. In R. Tummey & T. Turner (Eds.), *Critical issues in mental health* (pp. 161–175). Basingstoke: Palgrave Macmillan.

Webb, S. (2006). *Social Work in a Risk Society*. Basingstoke: Palgrave Macmillan.

Webb, S. (2009). Risk, governmentality and insurance: The actuarial recasting of social work. In H. W. Otto, A. Polutto, & H. Ziegler (Eds.), *Evidence based practice: Modernising the knowledge base of social work* (pp. 211–226).

Witkin, S. L. (2017). *Transforming social work*. London: Palgrave Macmillan.

Zedner, L. (2006). Pre-crime and post criminology. *Theoretical criminology, 11*(2), 261–281.

Emily Keddell

COMPARING RISK-AVERSE AND RISK-FRIENDLY PRACTITIONERS IN CHILD WELFARE DECISION-MAKING: A MIXED METHODS STUDY

Variable decisions are a persistent problem in child welfare decision-making. This article reports on the findings of a study of variability drivers in Aotearoa New Zealand. Using a mixed methods ecological approach, it compares 'risk-averse' and 'risk friendly' practitioners (n = 67 child welfare social workers). The study found the risk-averse group contained more non-governmental child welfare workers, but there were no other demographic differences. Risk-averse respondents were more certain of their conclusions even when little information was provided, and rated the children's safety lower. The risk-averse group estimated more harm to children over time, if there was no intervention. Both groups described risk and safety factors similarly, but despite this shared knowledge base, risk and safety level perceptions still differed. When explaining problem causes the risk-averse group focused on the past trauma histories of parents, whereas the risk-friendly group focused more on issues in the present. This pattern suggests practitioners conceptualise the meaning and weighting of risk factors differently, with some having a 'developmental lifespan- futurist' orientation as opposed to a 'welfare/needs-presentist' orientation. Implications for practice are discussed.

Decisions and risk

Decision-makers in the child welfare domain are frequently charged with assessing levels of risk that lead to decisions about children's care. In real-world practice contexts, assessing and responding to risk is contingent on socially influenced processes that shape perceptions of what constitutes risk, as well as considerable uncertainties about the outcomes of the available courses of action (Kemshall 2010; Munro 2010). Nor is decision-making simply about an individual decision-maker. Decision outcomes are shaped by interlocking factors across the ecological spectrum including social inequalities, political ideologies, policy orientations, institutional cultures and locations, policies and processes, group decision-making, risk assessment frameworks and available resources (Baumann, Dalgleish, Fluke, & Kern 2011; Bywaters 2015; Dickens,

Howell, Thoburn, & Schofield 2007; Fargion 2014; Fluke, Chabot, Fallon, MacLaurin, & Blackstock 2010; Gilbert, Parton, & Skivenes 2011; Hackett & Taylor 2014; Helm & Roesch-Marsh 2016; Keddell 2014a, 2014b). Nor do decisions occur neatly in time. They are often protracted affairs, or occur in incremental steps or as a series of related decisions also contingent on family and resource changes. In this complex social, temporal and material context, decision-making in relation to similar cases can be variable. While no two families are exactly the same, when statutory intervention or resource/service decisions are widely varied despite similarities in family situations or levels of harm, this creates a social justice problem. Serious intervention or access to resources should be undertaken in an equitable manner so as children and parents' rights are consistently upheld (Keddell 2014a).

While the wider ecological context is influential on decision-making, there are important influences on individual decision-makers that shape decision-making. These have been described in various ways: differences in practice wisdom, the professional discretion, analytical and intuitive thinking, knowledge use, heuristics, biases, role types, experience and value positions (Davidson-Arad & Benbenishty 2016; Enosh & Bayer-Topilsky 2014; Fluke, Corwin, Hollinshead, & Maher 2016; Helm 2011; Hennum 2011; Keddell 2014c, 2015; Munro 2011; Samsonsen & Turney 2016; Taylor 2016). This article reports some of the individual practitioner findings from an ecological mixed methods study that sought to answer the research question: what drives decision variability in child welfare in Aotearoa New Zealand? By splitting the respondents into two categories by their answers to an early survey question, two groups were created: risk averse (RA) and risk friendly (RF). By analysing both the quantitative and qualitative responses of each group, some insights were gained about important within-group differences within child welfare workers that may be contributing to variation in the perceptions of risk, safety and harm that inform decision outcomes.

Practitioner perceptions and decision outcomes

A number of studies have examined the relationships between values, perceptions of risk, knowledge use, and various demographic and individual level factors. Arad-Davidzon and Benbenishty (2008), Davidson-Arad and Benbenishty (2010, 2016) examined how practitioner attitudes towards child removal and fostercare influenced their recommendations to both remove and reunite children with their families of origin. By using a child welfare attitudes survey, the researchers were able to show that respondents' attitudes towards 'removal, reunification, duration of alternative care, and perceived quality of out of home placements' could separate them into pro-removal and 'anti removal' groups (p.107). They were then presented with a vignette and asked to give their decision preference. They found that the pro-removal group 'made higher risk assessments and recommended removal significantly more than the latter' (Arad-Davidzon & Benbenishty 2008), p.107. Križ and Skivenes (2012) compared workers' responses to an ethnic minority child in England and Norway, finding that the practitioners took either a child-centric or family focused standpoint when working with families. In a further study, they compared workers in Norway, England and California (Križ & Skivenes 2013). Using a vignette approach, they found Californians rated risk the lowest, followed by England and then Norway. Risk factors considered important also varied between the three national contexts. Workers in Norway assessed risk in a homogenous manner, while the other two had more varied perceptions of risk. They propose that differences are not only related to differing risk assessment practice frameworks, but also the child welfare system orientation, the uniformity or otherwise of that orientation, and level of commitment to a social democratic welfare state. They also considered how concepts relating to orientation translated into the frontline practice conceptualisation of important aims of practice, termed 'street level policy aims'(Križ & Skivenes 2014). They found that

> Norwegian street-level policy aims are child-centered and child welfare-oriented. English street-level policy aims are safety-oriented and child-centered; and US–American street-level policy aims are safety-oriented and family-centered, and that in the US., 'permanency' was understood as family preservation (p.71).

They also compared practitioners' views on domestic violence in relation to child welfare decisions as part of the same study. They found again that Norwegian workers considered the risk level to be significantly higher than the practitioners from England and USA:

> However, workers' justifications for and identification of decisive factors in the case are strikingly similar across countries. These similarities are observed for both high-risk and low-risk assessors, and they may exist due to widespread knowledge about domestic violence and its negative consequences across several countries (p.424).

This study highlights that in terms of knowledge use, a shared knowledge base does not necessarily reduce differences in risk perception and decision outcomes.

Fluke et al. (2016) in a US study tested workers on the 'Dalgleish scale' – one designed to test worker's position on a continuum from child safety to family preservation beliefs. By gathering demographics they were able to explore the relationship between a number of practitioner variables and their beliefs and values in relation to families. They found that more experienced staff were more likely to be oriented towards family preservation, whereas staff who had worked in the field for a shorter duration were more likely to be oriented towards child safety. This showed that practitioner attitudes and perspective do influence decision-making, as this demonstrated 'that child and family outcomes, such as maltreatment recurrence or out-of-home placement, are not solely determined by family and case characteristics' (Fluke et al. 2016, p.210). These studies highlight the interplay between personal values and beliefs, how risk is perceived or knowledge used to interpret risk, and national contexts.

Another element of interpreting risk relates to the concept of uncertainty – whether or not practitioners are able to make certain predictions in a context of unknowable outcomes and the fact that risk factors derived from correlation studies cannot be considered deterministic (Munro, Taylor, & Bradbury-Jones 2014; Parton 1998). An interesting question that flows from this is how practitioners respond to and use evidence in practice, and how decision-making tools such as consensus based tools or actuarial tools based on evidence of known risk factors are used in practice. For example, Gillingham (2009) found in a study of the use of a structured decision-making tool that practitioners subverted the tool to get the outcome they wanted. Others have found that whether people use consensus based or actuarial tools, they both have low to moderate interrater reliability, and neither are either very successful at predicting future risk of harm (Bartelink, De Kwaadsteniet, Ten Berge, & Witteman 2017). These studies show the gulf between practice tools and actual practice, and draw attention to the notion that even when stated knowledge bases and evidence for decisions are overt, that outcomes can still be variable. This is why a more expansive strategy for improving consistency that does not rely only on the use of a shared assessment tool is important (Keddell 2016).

Child welfare decision-making and the Aotearoa New Zealand context

Aotearoa New Zealand (ANZ) has a mixed orientation to child welfare services, both in terms of the traditional child protection/child welfare/child focused policy orientations, but also in terms of the state/NGO sector provision of services split (Gilbert et al. 2011). While similarly to other anlgophone countries it has had a basic child protection orientation, the legislation now 28 years old attempted to usher in child welfare ideals, at least in part due to the activism of Maori for more collective and preventive solutions to child protection. This attempt however was variable in its implementation and notoriously underfunded (Hyslop 2015). More recently, a strong child focused orientation has emerged, with the key tenets of children as individuals, child development, child trauma and future outcomes being the focus, all within the rubric of a social investment logic (Expert Panel2015). The increasing marketisation of child welfare services has led to a complex provision of services, with statutory services providing legal interventions, and NGO services providing generally support and therapeutic services. However, these lines are not clear cut, with some NGOs holding considerable legislated power, (such as being able to accept custody of children) and the statutory body (at the time of this study Child Youth and Family, but now the Ministry for Children Oranga Tamariki), providing some interventions such as family agreements and planning, and family group conferences, as well as now developing family services. Both employ predominantly social workers. The statutory agency requires social work registration or 'working towards' for employment. Mandatory registration is imminent.

A key feature is the presence of persistent inequalities in both system contact and outcomes of child and family services, with poorer people and Māori overrepresented in child welfare system contact (Bywaters, Brady, Sparks, & Bos 2016; Cram, Gulliver, Ota, & Wilson 2015). In terms of decision-making processes, the statutory agency relies on notifications from other professionals (many of whom are in the NGO sector) and Children's teams. The agency is a centralised agency with many site offices spread throughout the country. One aspect of the current reforms underway is in relation to decision-making, with the problem defined as one of children not being removed early to permanency enough, nor taking enough cognisance of child trauma. An additional problem identified in recent reforms was poor decision-making (Expert Panel 2015). A new practice framework was deemed the solution, but this has not yet been announced. All of these aspects make for a very complex decision-making environment, where the mixed policy orientation, system design, practice frameworks and logics, processes of reform and underpinning types of knowledge are multiple. Research into decision-making in ANZ is scant, although Keddell (2014c, 2017) found in a small qualitative study that child welfare workers in the NGO context tended to emphasise a strong family maintenance preference. Keddell (2017) also found that concepts relating to attachment theory were not used in a consistent manner when applied to decisions, and this resulted in some variations in relation to understandings of children's 'best interests'.

The study

This mixed methods study is based on a post-positivist epistemology, which emphasises methodological pluralism with a strong focus on pragmatic responses to the research question (Wildemuth 1993). Within this broad epistemological positon, it also draws on social constructionist concepts, as it attempts to examine the perceptions and decisions that practitioners make that emanate from the relationships between dominant discourses embedded in the social context and the meaning making processes of the individual (Rodwell 1998). In order to reflect both this and the decision ecology approach, as well as the exploratory nature of this study, two phases were developed. The first was an online vignette-based survey that elicits individual practitioner responses to a fictional case study. It gathers both scaled quantitative responses and qualitative data. Phase two consists of interviews and focus groups at three sites of the child protection statutory agency, in order to understand organisational arrangements, cultures and processes (Arruabarrena & De Paúl 2012; Stokes & Schmidt 2012). This article reports on some findings from the phase one vignette survey data.

Vignettes have a long history in the research of professional opinions, values, decisions and beliefs (Alexander & Becker 1978; Barter & Renold 1999; Finch 1987; Hughes 1998; Stokes & Schmidt 2012; Taylor 2006; Wilks 2004). They are established as the most effective way to measure quality of care in a health setting, as compared with standardised patient methods – considered the 'gold standard'. Of relevance to this study, vignettes in health research show that they are highly effective at capturing what practitioners actually do in practice (as opposed to their stated ideal practice), and at assessing variability in care (Peabody et al. 2004; Peabody & Liu 2007). The strength lies primarily in their ability to hold constant one variable – the case characteristics, – in order to establish variations in outcomes not caused by case differences. The vignette was written by the first author, then tested with two focus groups – one of statutory child protection workers, and one of NGO organisation workers. Small adjustments were made based on their feedback, particularly in relation to realistic levels of harm in relation to the thresholds for actions within the vignette. Particularly at the early stages of the vignette, the aim was to mimic the uncertainty of low levels of concern, and vagueness of information often present in first notifications. Vignettes should have enough detailed information in them to make the decisions asked of respondents reasonable, and should be as authentically recognisable to the respondents as possible (Hughes 1998; Taylor & Zeller 2007). The testing process helped establish these elements.

In order to mimic more closely the fact that in practice access to information about a family is not a one off event, but may consist of multiple, changing pieces of information gleaned from a variety of sources, this study used a staged vignette. At each stage, different types of information and levels of detail about the family were given, including some information from other professionals and some directly from the family. Each stage provided a more complex range of information and contained escalating concerns for the children's safety, from vague and low-level concerns, right up to serious disclosures of abuse from the children concerned. After each stage, respondents were asked to scale their perceptions of risk, perceptions of harm over time if nothing changed, what safety and strengths factors they see, and what decisions they would make. It also asks qualitative questions about what they considered to be risk factors, the causes of the family problems, what strengths or safety factors they see, and what goals they would prioritise in the case plan (Finch 1987; Hughes 1998; Križ & Skivenes 2013; Table 1).

Ethnic bias was also investigated in this study, by way of a split of the vignette into Maori and Pakeha families. These data are not reported here. After the four stages, additional qualitative questions were asked in relation to what types of assessment tools practitioners would use, how much time they would have to make a decision, who else had input into decisions, and what kinds of knowledge and ethical concepts they would draw on to help assess the case. Finally, practitioners' own views about how serious they felt the problem of decision variability is and what, in their view, causes it, were elicited. This is not reported here. Contextualising the vignette survey data within the organizational interviews and focus groups will enable an overall in-depth analysis that situates the perceptions and actions of the individual decision-maker within their ecological environment.

One area of interest that is fundamental to understanding differences in reasoning and decisions is differences in perceptions of risk. To attempt to understand this difference, respondents were split into two groups based on their responses at stage two of

TABLE 1 Questions asked at each stage of the decision-making survey

Quantifiable questions (either yes/no or likert scale questions):

Do you consider these children to be at risk of any type of harm?

Based on this information, how would you rate the level of risk of harm in relation to the children in this case?

How would you rate the level of safety of the children?

How would you rate the level of harm to the children over time if there was no intervention, and things continued as they are?

Do you think these children are currently being abused or neglected, and should be substantiated within the CYF system?

(If yes) How severe would you rate the level of abuse?

If the case had been referred to CYF, how close are you to 'forming a belief' that these children are in need of care and protection in terms of the definitions found in s14 of the Children, Young Persons' and their Families Act 1989?

Based on the information you have at this point, what would you do? (List provided)

Qualitative questions:

In your view what factors may be placing them at risk of harm? Please list. What additional factors are contributing to the abuse?

Apart from abuse or potential abuse, what other significant problems do you think this family are experiencing, if any? List

What is causing these problems? State both direct and indirect causes

What strengths or safety factors does this family show, if any? Please list

The family is investigated and a finding of substantiated child abuse is made. The family is referred for a Family Group Conference, and at the conference, a plan is made for the care of the children. While the plan is at least partially up to the family, if you were their social worker, what would you see as important goals of the plan? List the goals, and number them with 1 as most important the survey to the question: Based on this information, how would you rate the level of risk of harm in relation to the children in this case? This stage was chosen as it is when they were given some substantial information about the case, but the concerns for the children were still somewhat vague and the level of abuse was unknown.

Scaled questions and yes/no answers were produced as raw percentages in tables and graphs, and analysed for statistical significance using chi-square comparisons in SPSS. All chi-square comparisons used Monte Carlo simulation (100,000 replications) in order to counter the small sample size. Because the Monte Carlo simulation is a probabilistic method, this assists the analysis to cope with smaller sample sizes. The method's dependence on its inputs is a limiting factor inasmuch as the probability of the input's occurrence must be fair, but this also a strength as it means that the analysis does not need to rely on any assumed probability distributions (which may or may not be an accurate representation of the data) such as the bell curve (Cleophas & Zwinderman 2012). Decision outcomes were atomised in order to account for the multiple options available to the respondents, that is, each response was split into its component parts. Qualitative data was subject to content analyses through simple counts of items and phrases, then developed into more meaningful themes through inductive coding for dominant meaning patterns (Braun & Clarke 2006). While primarily inductive, some theoretical concepts were applied, particularly the concept of variability. This study was approved by the University of Otago ethics committee, the New Zealand Ministry of Social Development Research Access Committee, and went through the Ngai Tahu research committee consultation process.

Results

The table below shows the demographics of the participants in the first phase. Respondents were recruited from both the statutory provider of child protection services in Aotearoa New Zealand (Child Youth and Family), and all NGO services as defined by the relevant legislation (s396 of the Children, Young persons and their Families Act 1989) as either a child and family, Iwi or Cultural service. 67 participants completed the survey, and of these, 88% were women. In terms of ethnicity, 70% gave Pakeha, 18% Māori and 15% 'other' as their ethnic group response. The respondents consisted of a range of both Child Youth and Family and NGO child and family social workers, and represent around 5% of CYF workers. The representation of NGO workers is not known as the total is not known (Table 2).

From this total sample, in order to examine differences in risk perception and its relationship with other decision influences, as mentioned the respondents were then divided into groups in relation to their perceptions of risk at stage two, by their response to this

TABLE 2 Demographics of the total sample

Age range	22–69		Mean = 43	SD = 10
Holds a SW qual	Yes 90%	No 10%		
Entitled to registration	Yes 95%	No 5%		
Years experience	1–37 yr max		Mean = 13	SD = 9.2
Role type	CYF *n* = 46 (69%) NGO *n* = 21 (31%)		Total: 67	

question: Based on this new information, how would you rate the level of risk of harm in relation to the children in this case? Those categorised as risk-averse (RA) answered 4 or 5, that is, 'substantial risk' or 'high risk' ($n = 34$). No respondents answered 'not known' to this question. Those who were categorised as risk-friendly (RF) were those who answered 1, 2 or 3, that is, 'no risk', 'a little risk' or 'somewhat risky' ($n = 33$). It is recognised that labelling these groups as 'risk-averse' and 'risk-friendly' portrays them in particular ways for example, it could be argued that the term 'risk-friendly' gives negative connotations as someone who is careless or flippant, while risk-averse may also be construed as excessively cautious or overly interventionist. It may also overstate internal differences by implying dichotomization. It was difficult to find neutral terms, highlighting the influence of language on risk discourses in this context. Risk taking is similarly tarred with a variety of meanings from reckless to brave (Taylor 2017). The RA group had a slightly higher proportion of men at 15% v 6% (but n is very small). Ethnicity was broadly similar between the two groups, as was the mean age (43 v 42). Likewise, years of experience was similar at 13 years (mean) for both. Slightly more of the risk-friendly group held a social work qualification at 97% compared to 82% of the risk-averse group. The main demographic difference was in relation to role type, seen below (Table 3):

As can be seen, only 50% of the RA group were statutory child protection workers, compared to 88% in the RF group. These raw percentages differ from the overall split of 69%/31% of the overall sample. While this finding should be approached with cau-

TABLE 3   Role type of risk-averse and risk-friendly groups

	Risk averse %	Risk friendly %
Statutory child protection – Child youth and family	50	88
Non-governmental or community-based providing child and family services	50	12
Total	100	100

tion given the small sample size, it was corroborated by the overall finding that role type was related to risk perception overall, even when respondents were not categorised into the two 'risk' groups (Keddell & Hyslop 2016).

Perceptions of safety

The inclusion of questions in relation to safety was to examine the uptake of safety-oriented and strengths approaches in social work education and practice tools (Saleebey 2010; Turnell & Edwards 1999). Understanding if this influences practitioners' perceptions and decisions is important, given its aim is to balance the focus on risk and deficits child protection practitioners are so often charged with. In response to the question How would you rate the level of safety of the children? The safety perceptions of the two groups were most marked at stage two ($p = .02$) where for example, 55% of the risk averse group stated the children were either 'a little safe or not safe', compared to 25% of the risk friendly group. The significance of group membership (RA or RF) in relation to perceptions of safety declined over subsequent stages (to $p = .08$ at stage 3, to $p = .3$ at stage 4) (Figure 1).

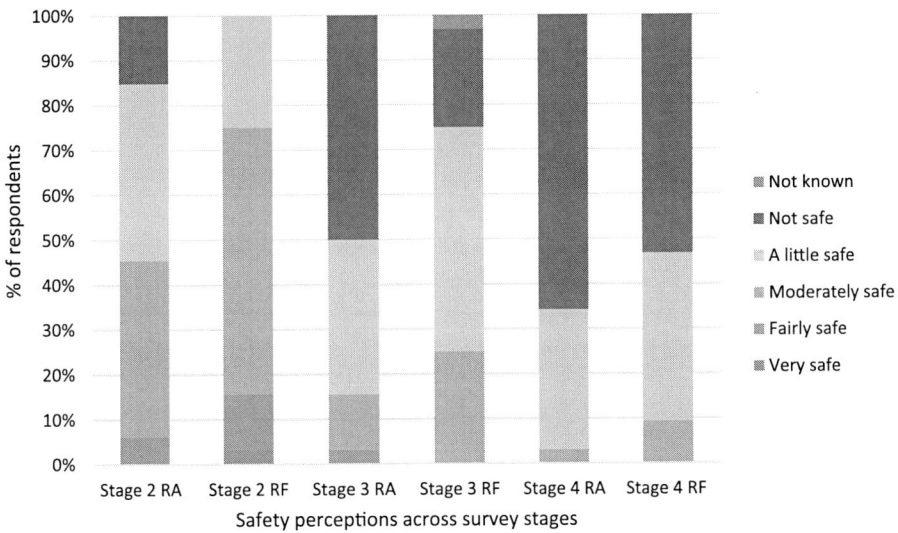

FIGURE 1 Perceptions of safety of risk-averse and risk-friendly respondents over stages 2–4

Perceptions of future harm

The most marked finding in the quantitative data was the difference between the two groups in response to the question: how would you rate the level of harm to the children over time if there was no intervention, and things continued as they are? This question was included in the survey to examine perceptions of the effect of the presenting problems over time into the future, as opposed to questions that examine risk perception in relation to the current situation. As practitioners are regularly making judgements in relation to both immediate and future outcomes, understanding how they conceptualise this in practice is an important element of decision-making, particularly in the child welfare environment where future uncertainty is a key feature of decision-making (Parton 1998). As can be seen in the graph below, the risk-averse group perceived the level of harm to the children over time as much higher than the risk-friendly group. The difference was much more marked than their differences in relation to current risk or safety perceptions (Figure 2).

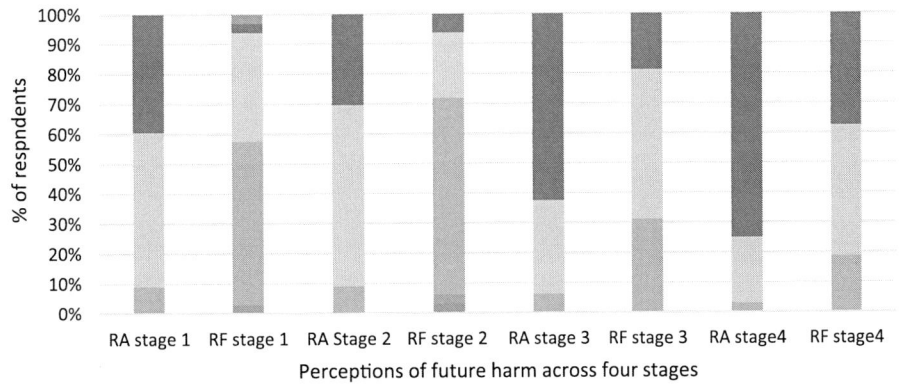

FIGURE 2 Perceptions of future harm by risk-averse and risk-friendly respondents across all stages

Tests for significance at each stage:

Stage $1 - p. = 4 \times 10^{-5}$, stage $2 - p = 1 \times 10^{-5}$, stage $3 - p = .002$, stage $4 - p = .02$.

Perceptions of abuse severity also differed between the two groups. Responses to 'how severe do you rate the abuse?' showed group differences, especially at stage two, where 74% of the risk-averse group gave 'fairly serious' or 'severe', compared to 46% of the risk-friendly group ($p = .035$). In response to the question 'how close are you to forming a belief', there was no difference between the two groups. This is likely influenced by the removal of the NGO practitioners from this group of respondents (who were overrepresented in the RA group), as it does not apply to their role.

Decision responses

The decision responses made by the respondents are difficult to analyse for several reasons, and although reported here can only be used to reach tentative conclusions. This is because the two types of child welfare workers – NGO and statutory child protection workers – were given different decision outcomes in the survey, as in real practice they each have a different range of decisions available to them. Because of this split, the numbers of RA and RF in each category are even smaller for each type of decision outcomes (those for statutory and NGO workers). In addition to this, respondents could tick more than one decision, as this again reflects real-world contexts where people may take a range of decision actions. Bearing these caveats in mind, examining the table below, which has n numbers left in to show small numbers, what can be seen are several differences between the groups who answered the statutory workers question. The risk-averse group at stage one are more likely to interview the children and refer to a children's team (a multi-disciplinary team outside of statutory services). At stage two the risk-friendly group were nearly twice as likely to recommend collecting more information from other professionals. At stage three, risk-averse respondents were twice as likely to hold a whanau hui (a family meeting at a level below that of the legally binding family group conference) and twice as likely to complete a child and family assessment, but surprisingly the risk-friendly group were three times more likely to complete a child protection protocol – a more investigative procedure than a child and family assessment.

Overall, as the child protection concerns described in the vignette increased and more detailed information was provided, perceptions of risk, substantiation, safety, severity and decision outcomes all converged to some extent, and more similarity between the two groups was observed. Perceptions of future harm however, remained markedly different.

Understanding the meanings beneath the perceptions: risks, safety, problem explanations and plan priorities

The qualitative data allow for further exploration of the issues of risk and safety perception, and enable a more nuanced examination of the between-group differences. After all, while descriptive differences are of interest understanding why these differences occur is important. In groups where there are few demographic differences (apart from role type), what else might be informing such marked differences in response to the same case? Practitioner underpinning knowledge bases, beliefs and values, the use of intuition or emotion have all been examined as possible contributors to decision reasoning and differences. As described above, influences such as child welfare attitudes, beliefs about problem causality and culpability, or whether the practitioner holds a child safety or family preservation orientation can influence reasoning and decisions (Benbenishty et al. 2016; Keddell 2011, 2014a, 2014c). Qualitative data help understand these aspects, as they can illuminate the ascriptions of meaning that respondents make that lead to differences in decisions.

In this study, to answer these questions, beliefs were examined in relation to: risk factors, safety factors, what is causing the abuse, beliefs about what is causing the family problems more generally, and asked respondents to describe their case plan and prioritise their goals for the family. Both groups identified similar risk factors and problems experienced by the vignette family. For example, at stage one when asked what factors may be placing the children at risk of harm, the following issues were given (see Table 3). At stage one both groups identified safety factors of a similar type and range, just as the risk factors were. When asked at stage two to note any additional risk factors, both groups identified disclosures of assault, lack of supports, multiple stressors, low parenting capacity, lack of sleep, financial issues and the fathers' learning difficulties. This suggests that practitioners were perceiving similar issues as indicative of risk (from across the ecological spectrum) – but weighting them differently in relation to risk and decisions. This is a persistent problem when attempting to rectify decision variability with common assessment frameworks or education about known risk factors as the problem is not lack of knowledge, but differential weighting of that knowledge (Bartelink et al. 2017; Skivenes & Stenberg 2013; Tables 4 and 5).

While the risk and safety factors identified were similar for both groups, when asked to describe the causes of problems, some differences were found. When describing problem causes, the RA group had a greater focus on the past histories of parents and psychological issues relating to that past, whereas the RF group was more likely to focus on issues in the here and now. For example: 'unresolved childhood trauma of both parents' was a typical RA comment, whereas an RF example was: 'Multiple stressors of finance, sleep deprivation, limited supports and options for independent changes'. Further qualitative analysis of the problem explanations showed that the RF group tended towards more tentative language in their identification of risk factors, where eleven out of twenty-nine responses of the RF group used language that was contingent, tentative or situational, either by saying a future outcome *may* happen, stating more information was needed before they could say for sure, or using words like 'potentially' or 'possibly'. For example, 'the children are potentially being exposed to domestic violence' and '… a possible indication of neglect (although more information would have to be gathered regarding this)'. Only three out of twenty-eight responses in the RA group used this type of tentative language.

Further differences were observed in the responses to the 'plan' question (see Table 3). The plan responses were split into child safety and family preservation codes, defined as follows:

Safety: where safety was defined as their first goal for the children, or removal was recommended, or that the children need to live in a 'violence free' home.

Family preservation: where their first goal recommended supports for the family, safety was viewed as achievable via family supports, or removal was specifically stated as a short term option until return home could be undertaken. Results were that for the

TABLE 4 Decision responses by statutory social workers at stages one, two and three, by risk averse and risk friendly*

Decision responses	Stage 1				Stage 2				Stage 3			
	RA %	No. of responses (n = 16)	RF %	No. of responses (n = 29)	RA %	No. of responses (n = 16)	RF %	No. of responses (n = 29)	RA %	No. of responses (n=15)	RF%	No. of responses (n=15)
No action	0	0	3	1	0	0	0	0	0	0	0	0
Collect more information from other professionals	63	10	69	20	19	3	38	11	27	4	14	4
Visit the family	56	9	62	18	38	6	34	10	27	4	21	6
Interview the children	56	9	35	10	31	5	31	9	20	3	38	11
Refer to an NGO/Community service	38	6	35	10	56	9	69	20	13	2	3	1
Refer to a Children's Team	44	7	7	2	38	6	28	8	7	1	0	0
Hold a hui-a-whanau or whanau hui	25	4	17	5	56	9	41	12	47	7	24	7
Complete a child and family assessment	50	8	41	12	50	8	45	13	47	7	24	7
Complete a child protection investigation	6	1	3	1	6	1	3	1	20	3	62	18
Hold a Family Group Conference	0	0	0	0	6	1	0	0	67	10	72	21
Try and negotiate a S139 voluntary agreement for care	0	0	0	0	0	0	0	0	13	2	14	4
Apply to court for orders	0	0	0	0	0	0	0	0	0	0	3.45%	1
Total responses	100%	54	100%	78	100%	48	100%	84	100%	43	100%	80

*All percentages rounded

TABLE 5 Reasons given for risk of harm, stage one, by risk category

	Risk friendly n =29	Risk averse n = 28
Neglect	16	19
Violence	30	24
Mental health	2	0
Developmental delay	4	7
Children's needs	11	7
Children's behaviour	7	8
Total	70	65

RA group, ($n = 30$), fifteen prioritized safety as the most important goal, and fifteen family preservation. For the RF group, nine were safety oriented, while twenty-two responses emphasised family preservation.

Discussion

This mixed methods study compares both descriptive statistical findings about perceptions and decisions between two groups of respondents who are described as risk friendly and risk averse, as well as qualitative data that may assist with understanding underlying concepts. The limitations of this study are: the small sample size which means the findings may not be generalisable; self-selection bias that may skew the findings; and the use of vignettes is not the same as real-world practice, so participants may give responses that differ from what they would actually do. Further research is required to establish how representative these findings are of the child welfare practitioner population. The splitting of the respondents into two groups is somewhat arbitrary and it may be that the differences between them are mostly explained by role type, although this is not known due to the sample size that precludes more complex analyses. The Monte Carlo analysis method relies on its inputs being fair.

Broadly, the main finding is that, as other studies have found, despite common case characteristics, perceptions of risk, safety, harm over time, and what decisions to take vary (Enosh & Bayer-Topilsky 2014; Taylor 2006). The staged study design using vignettes provides a unique way to show that variability in perceptions relating to decisions occurs even when the levels of harm and family characteristics remain the same, and how these perceptions change as more information is known. By separating respondents into two groups, more focus on what causes differences in perception can be examined. The RA group, which contained a greater proportion of NGO workers, rated safety as lower and the abuse the children suffered as more severe. They had a much greater belief that the harm to the children in the future would be severe if there was no intervention, and were more likely to refer to a children's team or interview the children early. It is unclear to what extent their heightened perceptions of risk, and future harm lead to more intrusive legal interventions. In the qualitative findings, there was considerable overlap between the groups' responses. Both groups gave similar descriptions of risk and safety factors, but when explaining the underlying reasons for family problems, the RA group tended to give more emphasis to parental histories of trauma, while the RF group was more focused on current stressors. The RF group was more tentative in their problem explanations, and emphasised that more information was needed to draw conclusions. In their plans, the RF group respondents emphasised the need for family supports, whereas the RA group gave more responses focusing on child safety.

From these findings, a nuanced and complex picture of those practitioners who tend to be more risk averse, and those less so, can be discussed. Even though the identification of risk factors and safety factors were broadly similar between the two groups, the perceptions of the level of risk, safety and particularly harm over time differed markedly, showing that despite a shared knowledge base in relation to risk factors, that perceptions of risk can still differ (Skivenes & Stenberg 2013). A nuanced analysis of the findings in relation to perceptions of harm over time (the most significant of all the statistics), the tentative and uncertain language of the risk-friendly respondents, the focus of the risk-averse group on historical trauma and more emphasis on child safety give a further picture of group differences. These factors suggest that the underlying use of knowledge and perceptions of the nature and effect of the children's situation shape practitioner perceptions of risk. The RA group showed more emphasis on the traumatic life histories of the parents and perceived future harm to the child as more severe and certain. This could be described as showing a 'developmental lifespan – futurist' approach underpinned by concepts from a child focused policy orientation (emphasising children's development and future child outcomes), trauma (emphasising the effects of past events for the parents and current events for the children as having a lasting effect on functioning) and risk factor science (emphasising the correlations of risk factors with future outcomes) – all of which brings a sense of certainty. The RF group could be described as showing a 'welfare/current needs' approach that is less convinced of harm over time, and more tentative and uncertain about the relationship between current events and future outcomes. This latter group had a higher rate of statutory workers, so this pattern may be more exposed to serious cases, and the mixed outcomes of fostercare, so that may also shape their perceptions. They are more focused on reducing stress to the parents through meeting concrete needs and education, and maintaining family preservation.

A developmental lifespan approach emphasises the impact of earlier trauma on parents and children and based on this knowledge base, makes assumptions about the future effects on children. This approach may incorporate the concept of multiple traumatic events, such as 'multiple adverse events', that can have a detrimental, cumulative effect across lifespan outcomes (Spratt 2012). The more present-oriented group may downplay the influence of trauma and the possible ongoing effects into the future. On the other hand, deterministic uses of risk factor science, and trauma and its related neuroscience knowledge base, have both been criticised for overstating harmful outcomes in policy and practice. In relation to risk factor science, correlations may be mistaken for deterministic causation, or as having effect sizes larger than they are. This can distort practitioner's thinking to overstate the risk of poor future outcomes, as well as making them appear more certain than they are. This problem with human decision-making has been identified for some time as one way in which humans overestimate base rates and effect sizes in relation to decisions (Enosh & Bayer-Topilsky 2014; Kahneman 2011). Munro and Musholt (2014) point out that many of the risk factors for child abuse are 'neither necessary nor sufficient', that is, no specific factor can predict abuse, and effect sizes can be small and mediated by a range of interrelating factors. The effect of abuse on the brain that may be underpinning beliefs about trauma and its effects has been roundly critiqued as overstating the emerging nature of brain science and the fact of brain malleability throughout childhood (Beddoe & Joy 2017; Edwards, Gillies, & Horsley 2015; Munro & Musholt 2014; Munro et al. 2014; Wastell & White 2012). The continuing debate into how risk factors and trauma should be responded to in practice is highlighted by these findings.

Conclusion

Much more research with a larger sample size is required to generalise these findings, but nevertheless they suggest that marked differences in risk perceptions exist between practitioners working in the child welfare field, and these may be related to a 'developmental lifespan-futurist' orientation as opposed to a 'welfare/needs-presentist' orientation. Understanding how these orientations can draw on similar knowledge bases but interpret them in differing ways, and how they may interrelate with values, beliefs and decision-making tools is a challenge for the future.

Supplementary material

Decision-making variability study – family vignette

Stage one:
A school has referred two brothers, Maxwell, aged 6, and Cody aged 5 to your NGO service, citing a general lack of care of the children. The school referrer says that the boys often arrive to school late, without lunch, and in clothes inappropriate to the weather. Other children complain that they smell. In terms of their behaviour and development, Maxwell is settled in school and learning well after an initially unsettled start. Cody has significant behavioural problems including hitting other children and regularly swearing at the teacher. He is developmentally delayed, with the speech and gross motor skills of a three year old. You find out that that there have been two call-outs by police to the house in the last 6 months for domestic violence incidents. On the second visit the children's father was arrested.

Stage two:
You visit the family, and meet the parents Shannon (25) and Dan (24) and discover they also have a younger child, Manny aged 2. They are Pākeha (*white*) OR They are Māori (*indigenous*) Shannon's mum is Pākeha and her dad is from Ngāti Kahungungu. Both Dan's parents are Māori – his mother is from Te Aupōuri and Ngāti Kuri, and his dad has a Pākeha father and Te Arawa mother (*tribal affiliations*). Dan lives for some periods in the family home but sometimes returns to live with his own parents, or travels away for seasonal work. His employment is casual so he ends up working about 6 months of the year full-time, for not much more than the minimum wage.

Occasionally he can get a month or so in the freezing works where the pay is much better, but it's not for long. Shannon works ten hours/week doing admin work at a local supermarket. Her mother lives nearby and often looks after Manny while she works, but he is in daycare for three mornings as well. They are struggling financially, especially as they have a car they bought on finance that Dan needs to travel to work, and the repayments are high. The neighborhood they live in has very few services for families and is unsafe at night as there are sometimes muggings in the local park. The one service they do have is a drop in for parents and young children that Shannon has visited a few times. Shannon seems relieved that someone might help her and is very cooperative. She says that she is constantly stressed with juggling the boys and work. She finds Cody especially difficult as he often runs off, hits the other children and can be very cruel to Manny. She can't leave him alone with Manny for this reason. He was born prematurely and still doesn't sleep well - he often ends up sleeping on the couch with Shannon as neither parent can get him into bed without a screaming match that wakes the other children. They are all exhausted as a result of this. Dan is somewhat uncommunicative at first, but comes around after a while. He says he finds parenting stressful, but tries to take the boys out fishing and to the park when he can. He says he sometimes loses it with Cody and has to put him in his room. When you raise the domestic violence call-outs, Shannon admits Dan and her often argue over the children, and this sometimes leads to him throwing things or 'shoving' her. The children are usually in the house when this happens. As she tells you this, she begins to cry. Dan gets up and leaves the room. Shannon is adamant that she loves Dan and doesn't want to leave him. She feels he has had a rough childhood and he needs her to get through life. She tells you a bit more about both their backgrounds. Shannon was an only child whose parents separated when she was a toddler, and then proceeded to have a protracted custody battle over her, ending when her father committed suicide when she was 12. She met Dan at high school and they have been together off and on since then. She finished school with solid grades, but got pregnant soon after leaving with Max and was unable to pursue tertiary study. Dan was raised by an aunt due to his own parent's alcoholism, but one of his aunt's partners was violent towards Dan for much of his middle childhood years, although after they separated things improved for Dan. He has dyslexia and has few qualifications. His aunt lives nearby and was helping with the children, but has recently developed diabetes and is housebound. Now Shannon and Dan try and support her as much as possible. At this point in the conversation, Dan returns to the room and angrily asks you to leave.

Stage Three:
After the last referral, a safety assessment was done by CYF (the statutory child protection agency), and as Shannon said that Dan had moved out, the case was closed. A month later, your NGO agency receives another referral about this family. Shannon has presented to mental health services with significant depression, and the nurse there has made a call (with Shannon's consent) given Shannon's distressed state and the way

the children presented when they attended with her. Cody destroyed toys in the health centre's play areas and Shannon vacillated between shouting at him and ignoring him, eventually becoming tearful and threatening to leave him there. You phone the school and the teacher says the children's attendance is dropping and when they do appear they are still often dirty, and smelly, although Cody has settled a little in school with the help of a teacher aide. Cody has twice mentioned to his teacher that 'mum and dad fight a lot' and one morning arrived at school upset and crying because of this. There has been another domestic violence callout by the police, as Dan had punched Shannon in the face causing a black eye and bruising. He has also broken two windows at their home. Shannon has taken out a protection order (a legal protection from domestic violence restricting contact) against Dan and he is currently living at his parent's house following this incident, although he is still frequently at the family home according to a neighbour you are also working with. You visit the family again but this time Shannon is uncommunicative, flat and uncooperative. She says she doesn't really want people 'poking around in her life' and states several times that Dan isn't living with her so there's not a problem as far as the kids are concerned. She has begun medication for depression, and been referred for counselling. She said she finds it a relief to talk to someone.

Stage four:

A month later, the school social worker notifies to CYF (statutory child protection agency). She reports that Shannon was seen hitting Cody in the school grounds after school by another parent. He was refusing to leave the school playground after school. Cody had pushed a younger child over and he was hurt, and so Shannon hit Cody across his legs twice. The next morning, the two boys are asked generally about about how things are at home, and both boys spontaneously state they are have been hit with hands and sometimes objects, by both parents. This seems to have happened on a few occasions over the last few months, but they aren't very specific. Cody has a mark on his leg from the day before. He also reports he is sometimes locked outside for 'a long time' as punishment, especially if he has 'been too rough' with the younger child. Once this was at night and he was very scared in the dark. If he wets the bed, he must change it himself and put the sheets in the washing machine. If he doesn't, he has to sleep in the wet and smelly bed. He wets the bed frequently, at least twice a week. They say Mum is 'crying and sad all the time', and that their parents still fight 'sometimes'. The children are also asked about what things they like about their family. Both boys say they like it on Saturdays when they all go to the park together and get an ice cream on the way home, they love their family dogs, and they like going to see their aunt because she 'always has lollies in her lolly jar'. Cody says he misses Dan now he has moved out but says there's 'not so much arguing now'. They also like staying up watching movies with Shannon on the weekends, and having popcorn and fizzy drink when their cousins come and visit. They also mention their neighbors often have them over to play with their own children and sometimes they stay there for tea.

Outcome:

The family is investigated and a finding of substantiated child abuse is made. The family is referred for a Family Group Conference, and at the conference, a plan is made for the care of the children. While the plan is at least partially up to the family, if you were their social worker, what would you see as important goals of the plan? List the goals, and number them with 1 as most important.

Explanatory notes in italics added.

Acknowledgements

Thanks to Dr. Ian Hyslop and Meran Campbell-Hood, University of Auckland for their helpful contributions on this project.

Funding

This study was supported by a University of Otago Research Grant.

References

Alexander, C., & Becker, H. (1978). The use of vignettes in in survey research. *Public Opinion Quarterly, 42*, 93–104.

Arad-Davidzon, B., & Benbenishty, R. (2008). The role of workers' attitudes and parent and child wishes in child protection workers' assessments and recommendation regarding removal and reunification. *Children and Youth Services Review, 30*(1), 107–121. doi:10.1016/j.childyouth.2007.07.003

Arruabarrena, I., & De Paúl, J. (2012). Improving accuracy and consistency in child maltreatment severity assessment in child protection services in Spain: New set of criteria to help caseworkers in substantiation decisions. *Children and Youth Services Review, 34*(4), 666–674. doi:10.1016/j.childyouth.2011.12.011

Bartelink, C., De Kwaadsteniet, L., Ten Berge, I. J., & Witteman, C. L. M. (2017). Is it safe? Reliability and validity of structured vs. unstructured child safety judgments. *Child & Youth Care Forum,* 1–24. doi:10.1007/s10566-017-9405-2

Barter, C., & Renold, E. (1999). The use of vignettes in qualitative research. *Social Research Update, 25*, 1–7.

Baumann, D. J., Dalgleish, L., Fluke, J., & Kern, H. (2011). *The decision-making ecology*. Washington, DC: American Humane Association.

Beddoe, L., & Joy, E. (2017). Questioning the uncritical acceptance of neuroscience in child and family policy and practice: A review of challenges to the current doxa. *Aotearoa New Zealand Social Work, 29*(1), 12–20. doi:10.11157/anzswj-vol29iss1id213

Benbenishty, R., Davidson-Arad, B., López, M., Devaney, J., Spratt, T., Koopmans, C., & Hayes, D. (2016). Decision making in child protection: An international comparative study on maltreatment substantiation, risk assessment and interventions recommendations, and the role of professionals' child welfare attitudes. *Child Abuse & Neglect, 49*, 63–75. doi:10.1016/j.chiabu.2015.03.015

Braun, V., & Clarke, V. (2006). Using thematic analysis in psychology. *Qualitative Research in Psychology, 3*, 77–101.

Bywaters, P. (2015). Inequalities in child welfare: Towards a new policy, research and action agenda. *British Journal of Social Work, 45*(1), 6–23. doi:10.1093/bjsw/bct079

Bywaters, P., Brady, G., Sparks, T., & Bos, E. (2016). Child welfare inequalities: New evidence, further questions. *Child & Family Social Work, 21*(3), 369–380. doi:10.1111/cfs.12154

Cleophas, T., & Zwinderman, A. (2012). *Statistics Applied to Clinical Studies* (3rd ed.). Various: Springer.

Cram, F., Gulliver, P., Ota, R., & Wilson, M. (2015). Understanding overrepresentation of indigenous children in child welfare data: An application of the drake risk and bias models. *Child Maltreatment, 20*(3), 170–182. doi:10.1177/1077559515580392

Davidson-Arad, B. & Benbenishty, R. (2010). Contribution of child protection workers' attitudes to their risk assessments and intervention recommendations: A study in Israel. *Health Soc Care Community, 18*(1), 1–9.

Davidson-Arad, B., & Benbenishty, R. (2016). Child welfare attitudes, risk assessments and intervention recommendations: The role of professional expertise. *British Journal of Social Work, 46*(1), 186–203. doi:10.1093/bjsw/bcu110

Dickens, J., Howell, D., Thoburn, J., & Schofield, G. (2007). Children starting to be looked after by local authorities in England: An analysis of inter-authority variation and case-centred decision making. *British Journal of Social Work, 37*, 597–617.

Edwards, R., Gillies, V., & Horsley, N. (2015). Brain science and early years policy: Hopeful ethos or 'cruel optimism'? *Critical Social Policy, 35*(2), 167–187. doi:10.1177/0261018315574020

Enosh, G., & Bayer-Topilsky, T. (2014). Reasoning and bias: Heuristics in safety assessment and placement decisions for children at risk. *British Journal of Social Work, 45*(6), 1771–1787. doi:10.1093/bjsw/bct213

Expert Panel. (2015). *Expert panel final report: Investing in New Zealand's children and their families*. Wellington: Ministry of Social Development.

Fargion, S. (2014). Synergies and tensions in child protection and parent support: Policy lines and practitioners' cultures. *Child and Family Social Work, 19*(1), 24–33.

Finch, J. (1987). The vignette technique in survey research. *Sociology of Health and Illness, 21*(1), 105–114.

Fluke, J. D., Chabot, M., Fallon, B., MacLaurin, B., & Blackstock, C. (2010). Placement decisions and disparities among aboriginal groups: An application of the decision making ecology through multi-level analysis. *Child Abuse & Neglect, 34*(1), 57–69. doi:10.1016/j.chiabu.2009.08.009

Fluke, J. D., Corwin, T. W., Hollinshead, D. M., & Maher, E. J. (2016). Family preservation or child safety? Associations between child welfare workers' experience, position, and perspectives. *Children and Youth Services Review, 69*, 210–218. doi:10.1016/j.childyouth.2016.08.012

Gilbert, N., Parton, N., & Skivenes, M. (2011). *Child protection systems: International trends and orientations*. Oxford: Oxford University Press.

Gillingham, P. (2009). *The use of assessment tools in child protection: An ethnomethodological study* (Phd). University of Melbourne, Melbourne.

Hackett, S., & Taylor, A. (2014). Decision making in social work with children and families: The use of experiential and analytical cognitive processes. *British Journal of Social Work, 44*(8), 2182–2199. doi:10.1093/bjsw/bct071

Helm, D. (2011). Judgements or assumptions? the role of analysis in assessing children and young people's needs. *British Journal of Social Work, 41*(5), 894–911. doi:10.1093/bjsw/bcr096

Helm, D., & Roesch-Marsh, A. (2016). The ecology of judgement: A model for understanding and improving social work judgements. *British Journal of Social Work, 47*(5), 1361–1376. doi:10.1093/bjsw/bcw091

Hennum, N. (2011). Controlling children's lives: Covert messages in child protection service reports. *Child & Family Social Work, 16*(3), 336–344. doi:10.1111/j.1365-2206.2010.00744.x

Hughes, R. (1998). Considering the vignette technique and its application to a study of drig injecting and HIV risk. *Sociology of Health and Illness, 20*, 381–400.

Hyslop, I. (2015). Elephant outing. Retrieved from http://www.reimaginingsocialwork.nz/

Kahneman, D. (2011). *Thinking: Fast and slow*. New York, NY: Farrar, Strauss and Giroux.

Keddell, E. (2011). Reasoning processes in child protection decision making: Negotiating moral minefields and risky relationships. *British Journal of Social Work, 41*(7), 1251–1270. doi:10.1093/bjsw/bcr012

Keddell, E. (2014a). Current debates on variability in child welfare decision-making: A selected literature review. *Social Sciences, 3*(4), 916–940. doi:10.3390/socsci3040916

Keddell, E. (2014b). Theorising the signs of safety approach to child protection social work: Positioning, codes and power. *Children and Youth Services Review, 47*(1), 70–77. doi:10.1016/j.childyouth.2014.03.011

Keddell, E. (2014c). Weighing it up: Family maintenance and children's best interests discourses in child protection decision-making. *Child & Family Social Work, 21*(4), 512–520. doi:10.1111/cfs.12168

Keddell, E. (2015). Constructing parental problems: The function of mental illness discourses in a child welfare context. *British Journal of Social Work, 46*, 2088–2103. doi:10.1093/bjsw/bcv096

Keddell, E. (2016). Is decision consistency in child welfare achievable without reversion to technical – Rational approaches?. *Visiting Academic, Child Welfare Inequalities Project*. Coventry University, July 14th.

Keddell, E. (2017). Interpreting children's best interests: Needs, attachment and decision-making. *Journal of Social Work, 17*(3), 324–342. doi:10.1177/1468017316644694

Keddell, E., & Hyslop, I. (2016). *First findings from phase one of the child welfare decision-making variability project: Research briefing paper*. Dunedin: University of Otago.

Kemshall, H. (2010). Risk rationalities in contemporary social work practice. *British Journal of Social Work, 40*, 1247–1262.

Kriẑ, K., & Skivenes, M. (2012). Child-centric or family focused? A study of child welfare workers' perceptions of ethnic minority children in England and Norway. *Child & Family Social Work, 17*(4), 448–457. doi:10.1111/j.1365-2206.2011.00802.x

Križ, K., & Skivenes, M. (2013). Systemic differences in views on risk: A comparative case vignette study of risk assessment in England, Norway and the United States (California). *Children and Youth Services Review, 35*(11), 1862–1870. doi:10.1016/j.childyouth.2013.09.001

Križ, K., & Skivenes, M. (2014). Street-level policy aims of child welfare workers in England, Norway and the United States: An exploratory study. *Children and Youth Services Review, 40*, 71–78. doi:10.1016/j.childyouth.2014.02.014

Munro, E. (2010). Conflating risks: Implications for accurate risk prediction in child welfare services. *Health, Risk & Society, 12*(2), 119–130. doi:10.1080/13698571003632411

Munro, E. (2011). *The munro review of child protection: Final report, a child-centred system.* London: The Stationary Office Limited.

Munro, E., & Musholt, K. (2014). Neuroscience and the risks of maltreatment. *Children and Youth Services Review, 47*(Part 1), 18–26. doi:10.1016/j.childyouth.2013.11.002

Munro, E., Taylor, J., & Bradbury-Jones, C. (2014). Understanding the causal pathways to child maltreatment: Implications for health and social care policy and practice. *Child Abuse Review, 23*(1), 61–74. doi:10.1002/car.2266

Parton, N. (1998). Risk, advanced liberalism and child welfare: The need to rediscover uncertainty and ambiguity. *British Journal of Social Work, 28*(1), 5–27.

Peabody, J. W., & Liu, A. (2007). A cross-national comparison of the quality of clinical care using vignettes. *Health Policy and Planning, 22*(5), 294–302. doi:10.1093/heapol/czm020

Peabody, J. W., Luck, J., Glassman, P., Jain, S., Hansen, J., & Spell, M. (2004). Measuring the quality of physician practice by using clinical vignettes: A prospective validation study. *Annals of Internal Medicine, 141*, 771–780. doi:10.7326/0003-4819-141-10-200411160-00008

Rodwell, M. K. (1998). *Social work constructivist research.* New York, NY: Garland.

Saleebey, D. (2010). *The strengths perspective.* Lawrence, KS: Strengths Institute, University of Kansas School of Social Welfare.

Samsonsen, V., & Turney, D. (2016). The role of professional judgement in social work assessment: A comparison between Norway and England. *European Journal of Social Work, 1–13.* doi:10.1080/13691457.2016.1185701

Skivenes, M., & Stenberg, H. (2013). Risk assessment and domestic violence – How do child welfare workers in three countries assess and substantiate the risk level of a 5-year-old girl? *Child and Family Social Work, 20*(4), 424–436. doi:10.1111/cfs.12092

Spratt, T. (2012). Why multiples matter: Reconceptualising the population referred to child and family social workers. *British Journal of Social Work, 42*(8), 1574–1591. doi:10.1093/bjsw/bcr165

Stokes, J., & Schmidt, G. (2012). Child protection decision making: A factorial analysis using case vignettes. *Social Work, 57*(1), 83–90.

Taylor, B. J. (2006). Factorial surveys: Using vignettes to study professional judgement. *British Journal of Social Work, 36*(7), 1187–1207. doi:10.1093/bjsw/bch345

Taylor, B. J. (2016). Heuristics in professional judgement: A psycho-social rationality model. *British Journal of Social Work, 47*(4), 1043–1060. doi:10.1093/bjsw/bcw084

Taylor, B. J. (2017). *Decision making, assessment and risk in social work* (3rd ed.). London: Sage.

Taylor, B. J., & Zeller, R. A. (2007). Getting robust and valid data on decision policies: The factorial survey. *The Irish Journal of Psychology, 28*(1–2), 27–41. doi:10.1080/03033910.2007.10446246

Turnell, A., & Edwards, S. (1999). *Signs of safety: A solution and safety oriented approach to child protection casework.* London: W. W. Norton and Company.

Wastell, D., & White, S. (2012). Blinded by neuroscience: Social policy, the family and the infant brain. *Families, Relationships and Societies, 1*(2), 397–414.

Wildemuth, B. M. (1993). Post-positivist research: Two examples of methodological pluralism. *The Library Quarterly: Information, Community, Policy, 63*(4), 450–468.

Wilks, T. (2004). The use of vignettes in qualitative research into social work values. *Qualitative Social Work, 3*, 78–87.

Laura L. Cook

MAKING SENSE OF THE INITIAL HOME VISIT: THE ROLE OF INTUITION IN CHILD AND FAMILY SOCIAL WORKERS' ASSESSMENTS OF RISK

This article conceptualises the role of intuition in professional judgement. It draws on findings from an empirical study of home visiting in child and family social work. The study used a psychosocial analysis of narrative interviews (n = 18) to investigate how workers constructed a professional judgement in relation to an initial home visit. In contrast to deliberative or analytic reasoning, intuition is defined as a non-conscious mode of reasoning, allowing the individual to reach a rapid judgement about a situation or person, often with striking accuracy. In this study, CFSWs' intuitions during their first encounter with the family were an important source of information for their assessment of risk – their emotional responses, 'niggles' and 'gut feelings' sensitised them to potentially salient information before it was rationally accessible. The study identifies five patterns used by Child and Family Social Workers (CFSWs) to assess risk during the initial encounter with parents: openness, coherence, emotional congruence, child focus and personal responsibility. It is argued that intuition is a product of experience, and is an important part of CFSWs' decision-making toolkit. However, when accepted uncritically, intuitive reasoning can represent a risk for professional judgement through the creation of bias. The article identifies specific biases relevant to judgements made on the basis of an initial visit.

Introduction

Everyday throughout the developed world, child and family social workers (CFSWs) prepare to meet new families, knock on doors and enter the private space of the family home. Their task during the initial visit is complex – they need to establish a relationship with the family, begin an assessment, investigate reported concerns and manage a sensitive conversation. Following the initial encounter, CFSWs must arrive at a judgement about what to do next (for instance, whether to close the case, to escalate concerns, to intervene or to conduct further assessment). Such judgements are often made in the context of time constraints, emotional pressure and high caseloads. This paper examines how CFSWs made sense of the initial visit, focusing on the role of intuition in professional judgement. The assessment process that follows a referral of concern is common across the western world (Samsonsen & Turney 2017). The findings from this study will, therefore, be relevant to child welfare decision-making across countries and settings where assessments are carried out.

Professional judgement

The concept of professional judgement has been a focus of international social work research. In the UK, this interest has been prompted by concerns around the quality of social work judgement. Research has identified a tendency towards poor risk assessments, descriptive rather than sufficiently analytical assessments and 'fixed thinking' and bias on the part of professionals (Brandon et al. 2009) which can lead to children being left at risk of abuse and neglect. There has been concern that the scope for professional judgement has been curtailed due to increasing regulation and administrative systems intended to increase accountability (Broadhurst et al. 2010). Comparisons have been drawn between the UK and other European countries, such as Norway, which appear to place a greater emphasis on professional discretion (Samsonsen & Turney 2017). A key question is how we can learn from the intuitive expertise of experienced workers, while remaining alert to avoidable biases.

The concept of intuition

Intuition is the process by which we come to know something 'without being able to explain how we know' (Vaughan 1979 cited in Topolinski 2011, p.275). It has been defined as a form of 'nonconscious holistic information processing' (Sinclair 2010, p.378). Expert intuition 'strikes as magical' when we see it in action (Kahneman 2012, p.11). It is sometimes described as a sixth sense, or gut feeling, that is later proven correct. For this reason, researchers have begun to explore the role of intuition in the diagnostic judgements of professionals, such as doctors, entrepreneurs (Baldacchino, Ucbasaran, Cabantous, & Lockett 2015) and most recently, CFSWs (Kirkman & Melrose 2014; Saltiel 2015).

In the psychological literature, intuition is defined in contrast to deliberation. Deliberative reasoning involves a conscious, effortful thinking process to reach a judgement. By contrast, intuitive reasoning is fast and non-conscious, with judgements experienced as occurring spontaneously (Kahneman 2012). The naturalistic decision-making (NDM) tradition conceptualises intuition as the product of 'large numbers of patterns gained through experience, resulting in different forms of tacit knowledge' (Klein 2015, p.164). The expert decision-maker has accumulated a rich and varied repertoire of patterns and is able to draw on these in order to make sense of complex situations.

In addition to experience, emotion has been recognised as a component of intuition (Sinclair 2010). From an evolutionary perspective, our emotional responses provide us with an immediate sense of whether we should approach or avoid particular objects or people before we are able to articulate why (Fiske, Cuddy, & Glick 2007). Emotional processes have been identified as crucial for the effective assessment of risk, our feelings 'efficiently and effortlessly' helping us to 'simplify complex scenarios and resolve ambiguity' (Finucane & Holup 2006, p.143). In relation to social work practice, Morrison (2007, p.225) suggests that the emotions of the social worker may act as 'deep level signals about information that demands attention' during assessment.

Intuition and professional judgement

What is remarkable about intuition is the frequency with which our intuitive judgements are correct. This is particularly true of social cognition. For instance, after viewing thin slices (very brief observations of a person's non-verbal behaviour) participants of psychological studies can predict intelligence, personality traits and even work performance with astonishing accuracy (see Topolinski 2011). It appears that reading people is an intuitive process which, at least at first-pass, is automatic and non-conscious.

In time-limited, uncertain situations intuition may represent an adaptive strategy. Over time and repeated experiences, individuals build up patterns that enable them to make sense of situations quickly and efficiently, without having to compare options (Klein 2015) or consciously consider all variables. In social work assessment, attempting to consider all possible variables and potential outcomes is likely to result in a 'combinatorial explosion' (van de Luitgaarden 2009, p.250).

However, intuition can lead to error. A series of biases have been identified in the psychological literature, including confirmation bias (the tendency to interpret information in a way that confirms our preconceptions) and credibility bias (the tendency to believe statements to be true if they come from a source perceived as trustworthy). Our social cognitions are also prone to bias; we tend to infer certain personality traits based on appearance, gender, ethnicity, perceived warmth and competence (see Fiske et al. 2007) which may lead to stereotyping.

In the UK, Munro (1999) has examined the operation of cognitive bias in social work judgement. Confirmation bias has been identified as a pervasive feature of assessment. Hypotheses reached early-on in the life of a case are unduly influential, suggesting that in terms of initial assessment, 'first impressions' tend to stick. Recent studies have focused on the 'front door' (Kirkman & Melrose 2014) or entry of families into social care services, identifying the use of intuitive decision-making in the processing of referrals (Saltiel 2015) as well as the potential for bias (Broadhurst et al. 2010) in the way that referrals are assessed. Credibility bias has also been identified as a risk in the processing of referrals, with the perceived reliability of the referrer being used as an intuitive gauge of risk (Regehr, Bogo, Shlonsky, & LeBlanc 2010).

There is, therefore, a danger that professional judgement might begin and end with intuitive reasoning, rather than representing genuinely reflective and informed thinking. Munro (1999) argues that professional judgement needs to utilise both intuitive *and* deliberative reasoning, the limitations of intuitive reasoning balanced by the strengths of deliberative reasoning (and vice versa). In this way, the risk of bias can be reduced. The present study explored the role of intuition (and potential for bias) in CFSWs' judgements in relation to a specific situation – the initial home visit.

The home visit and professional judgement

Despite concerns around the increasingly office-based nature of social work practice, home visiting remains integral to assessment in child and family social work (Ferguson 2016). During the home visit, workers need to offer support, ask challenging questions and confront the 'emotionally indigestible' (Cooper 2014, p.271) facts of child abuse and neglect. Ferguson's (2016) ethnographic work has identified some of the challenges posed by home visiting, including the risk of professional immobilisation in the face of overwhelming emotion. Despite a few exceptions, the home visit has been largely neglected within both the UK and international literature, remaining a hidden aspect of social work practice. It has been identified that the social worker's impression of the parent, particularly in relation to their perceived cooperation or hostility, may have an impact on CFSWs' assessments of risk (Hackett & Taylor 2014; Regehr et al. 2010). However, relatively is known about the way in which CFSWs make sense of their experiences during the home visit. How, for instance, do they select which aspects of their observations are salient? What signs do they tacitly regard as indicators of risk? How does their experience of the parent affect their assessment of risk?

The study

This qualitative research study used a psychosocial analysis of narrative interviews ($n = 18$) to investigate how workers constructed a professional judgement in relation to an initial visit.

The sample consisted of qualified CFSWs from two UK local authorities. At the point of data collection, both authorities divided front line children's services into Duty, Child in Need and Safeguarding teams. The interview sample included CFSWs from each of these teams. Duty workers featured more heavily (10/18) since they typically undertook a higher number of initial visits. CFSWs in the study had a broad range of experience.

Years in SW practice	Under 2 years	2–5 years	5–6 years	6–11 years	20+ years
Number of participants	5	2	5	3	3

Telephone interviews were undertaken with CFSWs immediately after they had carried out a home visit to a new family for the first time. The timing of the interviews reflected the need in the literature to investigate early assessment, as well as to capture workers' intuitive impressions. A narrative-inducing question was used: 'Tell me the story of the home visit you have just been on today in as much detail as you can remember'. Often workers were parked around the corner from the household they had just visited and the interview with the researcher acted as a debrief during which they organised their thoughts, impressions and emotions. Catching them at this point was crucial, since immediately following the home they were engaged in a process of sense-making.

CFSWs visited families for a wide range of reasons (see table below), often involving multiple presenting concerns (thus the presenting concerns total > 18). In two instances the presenting issue was unclear – due to this information not being provided during the research interview, or because the referral information was unclear to the worker at the point of referral.

Presenting concern at referral	Interviews
Children witness to domestic abuse and/or domestic dispute	7
Future parenting of an unborn child	5
Allegation of physical chastisement, abuse or assault	4
Child/Young person's behaviour at school	2
Child sexual exploitation	2
Young person at risk from community	1
Transfer-in from another LA	1
Unclear	2

As van de Luitgaarden (2009, p.255) observes, assessment involves 'story-building'. During the research interviews CFSWs were actively engaged in constructing narratives of the family to get a sense of their situation and arrive at a judgement. Psychosocial analysis (Clarke & Hoggett 2009) which makes use of narrative and psychodynamic theories, provided a framework for data analysis. The way in which CFSWs structured their narratives about the visit (including their pauses, hesitations and self-corrections) formed part of the analysis. Three themes were generated inductively from the data: sense-making (how workers generated hypotheses about need, risk and parenting capacity), self-regulation (how workers managed their own emotional responses during the home visit) and managing the encounter (how workers described directing the discussion during the initial visit). Interview transcripts were then re-coded under these three headings using NVIVO10, enabling further conceptual refinement. Intuition occurred at the intersection of sense-making and self-regulation – CFSWs often needed to manage their own emotional responses to the encounter with the family in the home (self-regulation). At the same time, these emotional responses often provided vital information in terms of their assessment of risk (sense-making).

Findings

Intuitive sense-making during the home visit

During the initial visit CFSWs were bombarded with sensory, affective, verbal and experiential data. They needed to make sense of interactions between children and parents, observe parental body language, examine the physical home conditions, consider which questions to ask and attend to the answers while ensuring that the family felt heard and respected. Understandably, families were often distressed at the prospect of a social work visit, so these tasks were often undertaken in a climate of distress, suspicion or hostility. For this reason, as one CFSW remarked:

> When you go into household you're heightened. Your expressions, feelings, emotions, your senses are all aroused.

During the home visit CFSWs described how people came and went, and how they themselves moved from room to room. Arriving at a judgement in the context of the initial visit involved therefore making sense of multiple social cues, rapidly changing situations and uncertainty. Within this context, the need to heed, and to unpick, one's intuitions was regarded by workers as crucial. As one CFSW cautioned, if 'you've got something in the back of your head you've *really* got to check it out!' Others gave examples of occasions when a 'bad vibe' which couldn't be articulated was later substantiated when more information about the family came to light. In the psychological literature, intuition has been described as the 'feeling of knowing' (Hogarth 2010, p.344). During the initial visit, workers' intuitive sense that something wasn't 'quite right', described by variously as a 'niggle', 'mental ping' or a 'gut feeling', allowed them to hone-in on factors that might be salient in terms of risk before they were able to say why. For instance, during one interview a CFSW repeatedly returned to a lack of 'flow' within the visit and her intuitive suspicion that something wasn't right in the home. The space provided by the research interview afforded her an opportunity to move from intuition to analysis – to reflect on her intuitions and what, if anything, they might mean. Another CFSW described a feeling of pleasure when watching an interaction between a mother and her young daughter, and his intuitive sense that the child was 'safe'.

Intuition has been associated with the ability to apprehend broad patterns in complex data (Klein 2015) as a result of prior experience. The ability to recognise patterns is an important skill for the professional social worker, particularly in identifying abuse (Taylor 2013). Workers' sensitivity to such patterns may become proficient given repeated experiences of working with families over the course of their career, allowing them to hone their intuitive capabilities. As one worker stated:

> It's about your own life experience, it's almost like your templates for life… I think for me it's a *gut feeling,* it's hard to explain - when you walk into a home - this is good, this is poor, or I'm not sure about this. I think that's your starting point, that gut feeling, or professional feeling… it's an unconscious thing … have I seen this before, or where have I seen this before and what was the result of that experience?

These eloquently termed 'templates for life', when drawn upon, allowed workers to quickly apprehend deviations to expected behaviours. CFSWs' intuitions, their 'gut feelings' and 'niggles' can, therefore, be regarded as an important part of their sense-making toolkit, developed through professional and personal experience. In relation to the initial visit, these intuitions appeared to act as an important starting point for assessment.

The role of pattern recognition in making sense of the initial visit

During the visit, CFSWs described inviting parents to 'tell their story'. What parents said in response informed workers' judgements in relation to parenting capacity and risk. I have used the term 'parental narrative' to refer to the 'story' told by the parent to the social worker (as described from the worker's perspective). CFSWs attended closely to what the parent said, as well *how* they said it. Five key patterns within the parental narrative were used by social workers to assess risk: openness, coherence, emotional congruence, child focus, personal responsibility.

·1. Openness

When making sense of the information presented by the parent, CFSWs drew on their perception of 'openness' as an indicator of risk. The perceived 'openness' of the parent (i.e. the extent to which they talked 'freely' during the visit, offering information with a minimum of prompting) appeared to be especially significant to social workers, and was mentioned by all of the CFSWs interviewed. Where CFSWs perceived parents as open they tended to come away from the visit feeling more reassured. For instance, one CFSW directly linked his favourable impression of the mother to his perception of her openness around sensitive issues:

Researcher: And what did you make of Mum?

SW5: Very good, actually. She spoke quite openly about the allegation. And again, she spoke openly about her family history.

A perception of openness could reduce the worker's level of concern even where the referral had indicated high levels of risk in relation to the child. For instance, one CFSW described how she was 'originally quite concerned' when reading the referral, yet left the visit 'feeling less concerned given that they [the parents] were quite open with me and told me quite a bit of information'. Workers were less reassured where they perceived the parent to be 'closed'. This was taken as a sign that matters were more complex or concerning. Openness acted as the worker's first-pass in relation to the parent, and was often treated as predictive of future parental cooperation. Where CFSWs perceived the parent to be open, they tended to leave the visit with a positive prognosis for the parent's engagement with social care services. This finding supports studies which suggest that perceived parental cooperativeness (e.g. in answering questions, providing information) is used by CFSWs to gauge risk (Hackett & Taylor 2014; Regehr et al. 2010). Most of the CFSWs interviewed were careful to balance their perception of parental openness with a consideration of wider factors, such as the case history and information from other agencies. However, in one research interview, the worker's perception of parental openness appeared to be the sole reason for the decision to close the case following the initial visit, despite a long history of similar concerns. There is therefore a danger that, when relied upon uncritically, this pattern may lead the worker to underestimate risk to the child and, potentially, to miss instances of disguised compliance. Since perceived openness led workers to a more positive first impression of parents, there is also a danger that service users who appear 'closed' may be unduly viewed with suspicion (e.g. those with English as a second language, anxiety or communication difficulties). Issues relating to ethnicity, class and gender may also lead workers to view parents as suspiciously closed when this may in fact be attributable to the power imbalance between worker and service user during the visit.

2. Coherence
When describing their discussion with the parent, CFSWs frequently referred to parents' ability to offer an account of their situation that 'made sense' and appeared to follow a logical structure. As one social worker said of a parent:

The things she said had flow – it wasn't as if she was jumping about all over the place, actually what she was saying and talking about *made sense*.

CFSWs appeared to associate coherence with parental competence. Parents able to give a clear account of their situation were described by CFSWs as 'switched on' and 'able to make decisions'. CFSWs' first sense of concern was often prompted by a break in the 'flow' of the parent's account – an intuition of incoherence in relation to what the parent was saying, i.e. that in some way it 'didn't make sense'.

One CFSW described a visit to a father who had previously lost a child to adoption. Part-way through listening to the father's account, the social worker described being suddenly struck by the fact that the father was unable to recall very recent, prior contact with his previous social worker. This intuition of incoherence piqued the worker's interest before she was initially able to articulate why. She described how she had experienced a 'mental ping' during this part of the parent's story. During the research interview, the social worker then began to subject this intuition to scrutiny – to consider why this aspect of the encounter with the parent had troubled her to such an extent. Moving from intuition to analysis, she began to consider different hypotheses that might account for the father's difficulty in recalling what she considered to be important information. He might, for instance, have memory difficulties or not wish to recall painful experiences. Or, more worryingly from her perspective, he may be seeking to deliberately withhold information. As a result, the social worker resolved to return to the case file to get a more detailed sense of the history. Intuitions of incoherence can act as a prompt for us to stop and seek further information. As Topolinski (2011, p.279) suggests 'we then become suspicious and begin to wonder, analyse the situation more thoroughly, and often discover the hidden cause for our discomfort'. For CFSWs in the study, experiencing a 'bad vibe' or a feeling that something 'didn't make sense' acted as a trigger for them to probe further. In this way, CFSWs' intuitions, their 'gut feelings' 'niggles' and mental 'pings' served to alert them to potentially salient information in terms of risk.

A coherent narrative may well be indicative of parental insight, ability and as an important way to gauge motivation for change (see Morrison 2001). However, it may be that coherence and logical thinking evident in the parent's account is not mirrored in everyday parental decision-making. The majority of CFSWs in the study expressed their intention to cross-check their intuitive impressions against other available information. However, in one instance a social worker's positive impression of a parent (as a result of her clear, insightful narrative) appeared to outweigh evidence of consistently problematic parenting behaviours. In this case, there appeared to be something of a 'halo effect' (Nisbett & Wilson 1977) in the worker's judgement; the assumption that their global evaluation of the parent (as coherent and organised) also applied to the parent's individual attributes (such as their parenting behaviour).

3. Emotional congruence

CFSWs attended carefully to the emotions expressed by the parent. Workers honed-in on whether the parent's narrative was emotionally congruent both in terms of their verbal account, and the type and intensity of emotions expressed. Firstly, CFSWs used the parent's emotional responses as a gauge of truthfulness, attending to the level of congruence between what the parent *said* and their accompanying expressed emotion. Workers described attending to body language, such as tenseness in the shoulders, 'fidgety' hands and other physiological indicators of the parent's emotions. However, as stated earlier, reading body language is a largely non-conscious and intuitive process that is consequently hard to articulate. As one worker stated 'I just got a *feeling* she was telling the truth'. Where the parent's emotions did not seem congruent or 'didn't match' with their verbal account, workers described investigating further, asking more probing questions and in some cases directly challenging the parent.

Secondly, workers considered the congruence between the parent's expression of emotion and the seriousness of the situation that had led to the referral. Workers attended to whether the parent was worried *enough* (whether there was congruence between the situation and the parent's emotional response and sense of concern), using this as an indicator of risk. For instance, one worker described feeling reassured that a mother 'was appropriately really angry' in relation to something that had happened to her child. In this instance, feeling angry (that one's child had been caused emotional distress) was regarded as an appropriate response from a protective mother. Conversely, CFSWs were more concerned when the parent's emotional response did *not* seem congruent. For instance, one worker described a situation in which the parent was 'saying the right things' and providing a coherent account of the situation, yet did not seem to be particularly distressed. The social worker herself had been quite affected by the details of what had happened to the children. When describing the home visit during the research interview, the worker kept coming back to the fact that the parent was not worried *enough* and tried to consider why this might be. 'Flatness' or 'despondency' in the parent's emotional response during the home visit was taken by some CFSWs as a particularly bad sign – indicative of a poor prognosis for engagement and lack of potential scope for change. This suggests that encountering someone who is depressed is overwhelming, instilling in the worker a similar sense of low mood and hopelessness. In these instances, there is a risk that the social worker's own emotional response to the situation might lead them to overestimate risk to the child and to underestimate the potential for positive change.

4. Child focus

The way that the child came alive in the parent's narrative had important implications for CFSWs' assessment of parenting capacity and their perception of risk. As one social worker summarised:

> It's what the parents are saying about the kids, the language they use.

Firstly, workers attended to the extent to which the parent was able to maintain a 'child focus' in their narrative, with particular reference to the child's experiences and emotions. Secondly, CFSWs were reassured where the parent's talk about their child was characterised by warmth and enjoyment. For instance, one CFSW observed that:

> She [The Mother] talked really warmly about the children... I asked about the children's favourite things to see what her view is of the children, and she talked warmly about the way they played ... she had a smile on her face and she was quite affectionate in the way that she spoke about them.

Conversely, workers were less reassured where they perceived the parent's description of the child to be focused on behaviour or problems, such as describing the child as the 'naughty one' among his siblings. The way that parents talk about their children may, indeed, be a helpful gauge of parenting capacity. For instance, the Working Model of Child Interview (WMCI) (Zeanah, Benoit, Hirshberg, Barton, & Regan 1994) measures parent's representations of their child. These parental narratives have been shown to predict parenting behaviour and quality of the parent-child relationship. CFSWs in the present study seemed to draw the apparently reasonable inference that an emotionally 'warm' or 'fond' description of the child was likely to be mirrored in the parent's day-to-day responses to their child. However, the majority of initial visits described by workers (12/18) involved them visiting parents alone. CFSWs would typically go to see the child afterwards, at school or college. Although CFSWs were very aware of the need to test the parent's account of their relationship with the child by interviewing the child alone, some workers expressed an intention to close the case without observing the caregiver and child *together*. There is a danger that parental representations of the relationship with the child may carry undue weight in terms of worker's judgement and, when not combined with direct observation of parent/child interactions, could lead to the underestimation of risk.

5. Personal responsibility

Workers attended to indicators that the parent was willing and able to take responsibility for their child's welfare. CFSWs looked for a sense of *responsibility* in the parent's account – that is, a narrative in which parents located themselves as a rational agent, able to make choices.

The parent acknowledging the 'concerns' about their parenting (i.e. the risks that had been identified in the referral paperwork), and their role in bringing about these concerns was viewed by CFSWs as an important first step in bringing about positive change. Social workers described feeling often reassured where parents demonstrated a sense of culpability, or regret, in relation to past events. For instance, a CFSW identified the following aspect of his conversation with a parent as salient:

> SW: He [the father] said 'if I had been more willing to consider what was being said to me, she might be in my care and not someone else's' … He's obviously given it some thought and shows some responsibility for his actions back then and some understanding of the consequences.

The social worker viewed the father's ability to identify his own role in past difficulties as key to assessing his future parenting capacity. In terms of initial visit more generally, CFSWs tended to be reassured by 'warm' 'amicable' and 'relaxed' encounters with parents, or where initial hostility or rejection (such as the understandable reaction to a SW visiting the home) was resolved throughout the course of the visit. The psychological literature suggests that the 'warm-cold assessment is the social perceiver's immediate "first-pass" as to whether the target individual (or social group) can be trusted…' (Williams and Bargh (2008, p.606). Given this general human tendency, CFSWs need to be supported to consider the role of their emotional and intuitive reactions in their judgements about risk, recognising both the value and limitations of intuitive reasoning.

Discussion

Intuitive reasoning played a key role in CFSWs' judgements relating to the initial visit, acting as a starting point for their assessment of risk. Their immediate emotional responses, or 'gut feelings' during the visit drew their attention to potentially salient information before it was rationally accessible. This appears to support the idea that emotion plays a crucial role in decision-making, and specifically, that affective intuitions are crucial in the assessment of risk (Finucane & Holup 2006).

Incoherence intuitions, or the 'instantaneous feeling of whether something makes sense or is wrong or inconsistent' (Topolinski 2011, p.277) were key to making sense of the initial visit. An intuition of incoherence in relation to the parent's account – a sense that something wasn't quite right – acted as a prompt for further investigation. However, this perhaps suggests a risk that CFSWs could be too readily persuaded by an open, consistent and congruent account of family life.

Expert intuition has been conceptualised as involving experience and pattern recognition (Klein 2015). It may be that workers' sensitivity to such patterns becomes proficient given repeated experiences of working with families. As one CFSW described, personal and professional experience may provide workers with 'templates' allowing them to quickly spot deviations to expected behaviours. Intuitive reasoning may, therefore, have much in common with the concept of practice wisdom.

What was striking during the research interviews was the differing extent to which individual CFSWs subjected their intuitive responses to scrutiny. Most workers spoke of their intention to seek further information to verify or disconfirm their intuitions, while a minority expressed a fixed judgement following the visit. Perhaps what is crucial for the effective use of intuition (and avoidance of bias) is the extent to which CFSWs subject their intuitions to critical scrutiny, using them as a starting point (rather than an end-point) for judgement.

Caution should be exercised in generalising from these findings to *all* home visits, since the initial visit represented a particularly focused type of assessment which may not be typical in the context of longer term assessment and intervention. This paper has focused in detail on how CFSWs made sense of a particular aspect of the visit – the parental narrative – in order to demonstrate how intuition contributes to professional judgement. However, other aspects of the social worker's observations such as the home conditions and interactions between carers, were also subject to similar intuitive sense-making processes.

This study examined CFSWs' perspectives on the home visit. Families are likely to have quite different experiences and views of what is important. In offering an account of home visiting from the perspective of the social worker, this research regarded as complementary to studies (e.g. Platt 2008) which have explored service users' perceptions of assessment.

Implications for practice

The findings from this study suggest that we need to acknowledge the value of affective and intuitive aspects of social work decision-making, while remaining alert to predictable biases. One way CFSWs can do this is to attempt to subject their judgements to critical scrutiny; to try to trace back the reasoning and the 'shortcuts' they may have used. Many workers in the study began this process during the research interview, exploring their thinking and considering how their intuitive responses may have shaped their judgement. The findings of this paper offer a framework through which CFSWs might begin this process – to consider how their intuitive impressions of the parent may have influenced their perception of risk. The five patterns identified in this paper could form the basis of a reflective aid for use in supervision, especially necessary where workers are managing complex, high caseloads.

If intuitive expertise draws on prior experience (Klein 2015) and learning then it follows that 'intuition can be educated' if individuals are supported to 'learn the 'right' lessons from the interactions with the world' (Hogarth 2010, p.248). To develop their intuition, CFSWs need to know the results of previous decisions they have made. Given the inherent uncertainty involved in social work judgements, we cannot say whether they were 'correct' but it may be useful for SWs to know the outcome. To find out, for instance, whether a case closed following an initial visit was re-opened a week later. The findings of this study support Kirkman and Melrose's (2014) conclusion that feedback loops could be a valuable feature of assessment teams.

The research interviews gave CFSWs a space for reflection – an opportunity to move from intuition to analysis. Interpersonal spaces, including supervision and the social work office (Saltiel 2015) provide similar opportunities for reflection. Although reflective practice is widely regarded as valuable, within the context of financial austerity supervision and support for reflection is often threatened by time constraints. This study suggests that reflection in social work is essential for effective professional judgement – CFSWs need to be supported to subject their judgements to scrutiny on both an individual and organisational level. If they do not, the risk of bias increases along with the risk to the children and families subject to their decisions.

Conclusion

Arriving at a professional judgement in relation to the initial visit involves the integration of sensory, intuitive, emotional and relational information. This is complex, skilled and demanding work, requiring workers to draw on their personal and practice experience. Intuition has been identified as an important part of CFSWs' sense-making toolkit. Workers' intuitions alerted them to potentially salient information amongst the innumerable data presented to them during the visit. This study has identified some of the risks for professional judgement when CFSWs 'gut feelings' are not subjected to reflection. However, it should be noted that most CFSWs in the study appeared to use their intuitions as a starting point, rather than an end-point for their professional judgement. Professional intuitions are perhaps best regarded as hypotheses to be tested. In terms of social work judgement, this means using intuition as an aid, rather than substitute for, analysis.

References

Baldacchino, L., Ucbasaran, D., Cabantous, L., & Lockett, A. (2015). Entrepreneurial research on intuition: A critical analysis and research agenda. *International Journal of Management Reviews, 17*, 212–231.

Brandon, M., Bailey, S., Belderson, P., Gardner, R., Sidebotham, P., & Dodsworth, J. (2009). *Understanding serious case reviews and their impact: A biennial analysis of serious case reviews 2005–2007*. London: Department for Children, Schools and Families.

Broadhurst, K., Wastell, D., White, S., Hall, C., Peckover, S., Thompson, K., … Davey, D. (2010). Performing 'initial assessment': Identifying the latent conditions for error at the front-door of local authority children's services. *British Journal of Social Work, 40*(2), 352–370.

Clarke, S., & Hoggett, P. (2009). *Researching beneath the surface: Psycho-social research methods in practice*. London: Karnac.

Cooper, A. (2014). A short psychosocial history of British child abuse and protection: Case studies in problems of mourning in the public sphere. *Journal of Social Work Practice, 28*(3), 271–285.

Ferguson, H. (2016). Researching social work practice close up: Using ethnographic and mobile methods to understand encounters between social workers, children and families. *British Journal of Social Work, 46*(1), 153–168.

Finucane, M., & Holup, J. (2006). Risk as value: Combining affect and analysis in risk judgments. *Journal of Risk Research, 9*(2), 141–164.

Fiske, S., Cuddy, A., & Glick, P. (2007). Universal dimensions of social cognition: Warmth and competence. *Trends in Cognitive Sciences, 11*(2), 77–83.

Hackett, S., & Taylor, A. (2014). Decision making in social work with children and families: The use of experiential and analytical cognitive processes. *British Journal of Social Work, 44*(8), 2182–2199.

Hogarth, R. (2010). Intuition: A challenge for psychological research on decision making. *Psychological Inquiry, 21*(4), 338–353.

Kahneman, D. (2012). *Thinking, fast and slow*. London: Penguin.

Kirkman, E., & Melrose, K. (2014). *Decision-making in children's social work: An analysis of the 'front door' system*. London: Department for Education.

Klein, G. (2015). A naturalistic decision making perspective on studying intuitive decision-making. *Journal of Applied Research in Memory and Cognition, 4*, 164–168.

Morrison, T. (2001). Assessment of parental motivation to change. In J. Horwath (Ed.), *The child's world*. London: Jessica Kingsley.

Morrison, T. (2007). Emotional intelligence, emotion and social work: Contexts, characteristics, complications and contribution. *British Journal of Social Work, 37*(2), 245–263.

Munro, E. (1999). Common errors of reasoning in child protection work. *Child Abuse and Neglect, 23*(8), 745–758.

Nisbett, R., & Wilson, T. (1977). The Halo effect: Evidence for unconscious alteration of judgements. *Journal of Personality and Social Psychology, 35*(4), 250–256.

Platt, D. (2008). Care or control? The effects of investigations and initial assessments on the social worker–parent relationship. *Journal of Social Work Practice, 22*(3), 301–315.

Regehr, C., Bogo, M., Shlonsky, A., & LeBlanc, V. (2010). Confidence and professional judgment in assessing children's risk of abuse. *Research on Social Work Practice, 20*(6), 621–628.

Saltiel, D. (2015). Observing front line decision making in child protection. *British Journal of Social Work, 46*(7), 2104–2119.

Samsonsen, V., & Turney, D. (2017). The role of professional judgement in social work assessment: A comparison between Norway and England. *European Journal of Social Work, 20*(1), 112–124.

Sinclair, M. (2010). Misconceptions about intuition. *Psychological Inquiry, 21*(4), 378–386.

Taylor, B. (2013). *Professional decision making and risk in social work*. London: Sage.

Topolinsky, S. (2011). A process model of intuition. *European Review of Social Psychology,* *22*(1), 274–315.

van de Luitgaarden, G. (2009). Evidence-based practice in social work: Lessons from judgment and decision-making theory. *British Journal of Social Work, 39*(2), 243–260.

Williams, L., & Bargh, J. (2008). Experiencing physical warmth promotes interpersonal warmth. *Science, 322*(5901), 606–607.

Zeanah, C., Benoit, D., Hirshberg, L., Barton, M., & Regan, C. (1994). Mother's representations of their infants are concordant with infant attachment classifications. *Developmental Issues in Psychiatry and Psychology, 1*, 9–18.

Peter Hall

MENTAL HEALTH ACT ASSESSMENTS – PROFESSIONAL NARRATIVES ON ALTERNATIVES TO HOSPITAL ADMISSION

This article draws on themes derived from research conducted as part of a doctoral study, using Framework Analysis, in which fifteen mental health professionals were involved in nine Mental Health Act assessments in the UK. In this work, risk is explored in terms of the social context, using a social constructionist perspective, in which concepts of 'social crisis / mental illness', professional negotiations and social capital are explored. The key findings highlighted: the social constructions of service users' worlds, as presented by the Approved Social Workers (ASWs) and Home Treatment Professionals (HTPs), were notably different; the negotiations between the ASWs and HTPs provided the ASWs with a number of roles including negotiator, deal-maker and decision-maker; and the service user's social network and the provision of home treatment showed that the 'treatments' provided can be seen as a shared role. Finally, the implications for contemporary mental health social work practice are presented.

Introduction: the special case of mental health act assessments

For many years, and even more so today, being assessed under the Mental Health Act (MHA) has been seen by many professionals as a precursor to compulsory hospital admission. This type of assessment, in the UK, has occupied such an invidious place in both professional and public imagination that the association between MHA assessments and being 'sectioned' is now well entrenched in popular myth (Barnes 1990).

The role of the MHA assessor (previously undertaken by an Approved Social Worker [ASW], but now by an Approved Mental Health Professional [AMHP]) has been seen as problematic due to the multiplicity of the role's dimensions, which inevitably creates uncertainty (Golightley 2014; Kinney 2010). These uncertainties are present in both professional and lay discourses. The AMHP is expected to have significant knowledge and skills in mental health work and to exercise 'independent judgement and be personally accountable for his own practice...' (Golightley 2014, p.71). Central to exercising independent judgement is the need to use a significant skill set to be able to engage with 'patients' and be able to explore the social context in which the assessment is undertaken.

MHA assessors 'have a wider role than that of doctors... having regard to any wishes expressed by relatives and any other circumstances...' during the assessment (Barber, Brown, & Martin 2012, p.9). What characterises an assessor in the assessment process is their ability to recognise and 'address some of the key issues relating to risks, rights... the centrality of values and ethics in implementing mental health law' (Coppock & Dunn 2010, p.63).

One reason why MHA assessments are so little understood is the fact that there is paucity of research in this area (Campbell 2010; Sheppard 1990). Despite some studies which have indicated connections [for example, between community provision and assessment outcomes (Dunn 2001) and social capital and assessment outcomes (Quirk, Lelliott, Audini, & Buston 2003)], findings which propose not only psychological factors (Davidson & Campbell 2010; Gregor 2010) but also factors which include local resources, social networks and professional norms are significant. As such, there remains a mystery around MHA assessments which continues to be viewed as something which cannot be understood or explained.

Researchers suggest that hospital admissions are often associated with a lack of community resources, home treatment teams, support from families and poor communication between professionals (Barnes 1990; Booth et al. 1985; Bowl, Barnes, & Fisher 1987; Fisher, Barnes, & Bowl 1987). Although it is not unusual for professionals to interpret MHA assessment outcomes in terms of a biological condition which needs hospital treatment, this understanding is usually constructed within a culture where sovereignty of the medical model is not fully subjected to critical examination.

> A candidate patient's chance of being sectioned is likely to increase when there are no realistic alternatives to in-patient care. This typically occurs when staff have insufficient time to set such alternatives in place and are unsupported by other professionals in doing this (Quirk et al. 2003, p.119)

The traditional understanding of an MHA assessment equating to being 'sectioned' (Barnes, Bowl, & Fisher 1990) is often not addressed within contemporary health care settings, with alternative assessment outcomes and treatments remaining unexplored. With increasing numbers of Mental Health detentions taking place year-on-year (CQC 2014), many people now live with the experience of being 'sectioned' and the consequences of being so labelled. The continuing increase in detentions under the MHA, together with the increasing number of people with mental health problems in many industrial countries, would suggest that changes to community healthcare are urgently required.

Hall (1995); Hall (2015) argues that the role of the social worker complements that of other medical professionals when using the medical model alongside a social constructionist model of care (Tew 2005). Here, all of the circumstances are considered and patients and their families are encouraged to identify the precipitating reasons for their crisis, rather than viewing MHA assessments simply as a 'mental health' problem. Essentially, this involves incorporating a wider range of concepts, such as seeing the patient as an asset, social capital and reciprocity (Cahn 2000). There is a need for utilising these concepts to broaden the assessment process, thus helping to counteract the more restrictive views of the dominant medical perspective.

So the question arises as to how we should respond to the changing nature of mental illness in Western society, and what theories of understanding are available to us to help develop practice with people who are assessed under the MHA?

Literature review

Through listening to the assessors' stories of MHA assessments and from a review of the research on MHA assessments and home treatment, three major concepts are identified which may enhance practitioners' understanding of their practice; these being: home treatment, professional decision-making and practice models.

Home treatment

The concept of treatment in the community (home treatment) was introduced into discourse through the National Service Framework for Mental Health (DoH 1999) policy, whereby 24 h access to emergency teams became available. Guidance on the use of home treatment and the MHA was made clear in the Department of Health's policy guidance (DoH 2001) and as a framework to understand the value of such teams (Johnson 2004).

Booth et al. (1985) were amongst the earliest researchers of the MHA, identifying and exploring crisis services as an alternative to hospital admission. They explored how crisis teams (home treatment) can work with ASWs to provide an effective service, identifying three broad levels of collaboration where this can take place: strategic, operational and practitioner. They viewed the issue of resources as central. 'One fifth of all hospital admissions were felt, by the social worker, to have been avoidable given a reasonable level of provision of alternative services' (Booth et al. 1985, p.79). Avoidable admissions were seen in part as being problems of collaboration, which fall into three categories: problems of access, problems of attitude or relationships, and problems of procedure.

Problems of access: This was understood by Booth et al. simply in terms of difficulties of co-ordination or people not being available. The unpredictable nature of psychiatric crises does not always coincide with professional schedules. These problems were seen as inevitable, but also seen to be 'exacerbated by working routines, professional methods and personal idiosyncrasies of manner, style and approach' (Booth et al. 1985, p.81).

Problems of attitude or relationships: Booth et al. (1985) identified these in terms of friction and conflict between social workers and doctors, drawing on Huntington's (1981) 'two cultures' theory. Huntington explores the differences between social work and general medical practice, identifying that there are marked differences of 'knowledge, learned values, standards, technology, technique, work orientation, language, identity and relational orientations' (Huntington 1981, p.73). It was seen that different 'perceptions of each other's role and responsibilities, in their interpretation of the nature and gravity of the crisis, or in their views as to what is to be done' (Huntington 1981, p.82) all contributed to the assessment outcome.

Problems of procedure: Huntington (1981, p.84) identified that 'impaired collaboration' was caused by breakdowns in communication at an organisational level and by failures to apply proper procedures due to unclear 'administrative divisions of functions, powers and responsibilities between the health and social services'. These problems arose around the differing interpretations of the MHA and clinical responsibilities. Like Huntington, Langan (1989) suggests that the timescale in which assessments have to be completed is problematic, with restricted opportunities to 'step back', similar to Schon's (1987) 'reflection-in action', and having insufficient time allocated for decision-making. This need to step back refers to ASWs being able to reflect on their practice and assessing whether they can justify and explain the reasons for hospital detention. Langan also suggests that the lack of alternative provisions is not the only factor which influences ASWs when using compulsory powers. The ASWs in this study did not always have a clear understanding of what was required of them and their practice in terms of their 'social, legal and ethical as well as medical considerations' (Langan 1989, p.1). The ASWs had no clearly-established patterns of assessment or good models of practice.

Analysis of the literature on home treatment aids our understanding of the issues around community provision for assessors involved in MHA assessments and provides a discussion framework in this underdeveloped area of practice. Home treatment support, as part of the assessment process can, under the right conditions, complement a narrow medical focus on 'mental disorders' and present an opportunity to broaden our understanding of the assessment process to include social networks and the positive contribution that a patient brings to the assessment process and, as such, supports individuals to manage better the psychosocial consequences of their diagnosis.

Professional decision-making

Langan (1989) has documented the ability of ASWs to look at alternatives to hospital admission. He reports that they feel unable to 'gain clarity' around the decision-making process, feeling that their only choice when undertaking assessments is between 'compulsory admission and allowing the status quo to continue' (Langan 1989, p.170). An ASW's ability to make decisions can be seen as a key area for investigation, with each assessment having its own unique circumstances and characteristics. Decisions made by assessors can have fundamental and groundbreaking consequences on patients' lives; consequently, assessors are held personally accountable for their practice. For Langan, there seem to be some 'relatively easy' alternatives to hospital provision readily available but remaining unused, 'such as temporary removal from family members, or moving the individual to a home for the elderly or use of family aides could have been and were not used' (Langan 1989, p.170). However, Langan does not seem to take account of the rituals which mark the assessment process, the negotiations which have to take place between professionals who may have very different practice philosophies and the consequences of challenging the established orthodoxy.

Peay (2003), following Sheppard (1990), further explores the decision-making styles adopted by professionals undertaking MHA assessments. Peay's research uses a single case study to gain assessors' views, in which she examines their philosophical styles, decision-making and recommended courses of action. The case study:

...concerned a psychiatrist and an ASW visiting a young black patient, Robert Draper, who was previously known to the service and about whom there had been complaints by his neighbours. There was evidence to suggest that the patient might be psychotic; the patient refused admission to hospital for assessment or treatment (Peay 2003, p.187)

The participants, forty paired assessors (one medical consultant and one social worker) were asked to review the case study and make recommendations as to which treatment course of action they would follow and why they chose hospital or community outcomes. Paired assessors were asked which role's description best described their practice - clinical, legal or ethical.

Clinical decision-maker: ...someone who was essentially driven by what was in the patient's and/or society's **best interests**, who looked to the Act only to determine whether there were legal powers that could be invoked in order to pursue these prior best interests

Legal decision-maker: ...was someone who carried around, either literally or metaphorically, an awareness of their **legal powers** and duties under the Act, together with the framework of safeguards it provides for patients, and allowed predominantly these factors to drive their decision-making

Ethical decision-maker: ...was one driven by questions of **capacity**. Was the patient capable of deciding for him/herself? Only if the person lacked capacity would the psychiatrist or ASW look either or both to best interests and/or to the Act. Hence, only incapacity would trigger interventions against the patient's objection (Peay 2003, p.187) [emboldment added]

The majority of the social workers and consultants, as paired decision-makers, see themselves in the 'clinical decision-maker' role, with only six social workers having no allegiance to just one model. For Peay, these types of decision-makers are not seen as having dogmatic views, but rather they are open to negotiations and, as such, negotiations can refocus the narrative and 'labelling' of the service user. As a result of the predominate clinical role taken by the social workers, the medical perspective was seen as paramount, with less credence given to the social context in which the service users found themselves.

An exploration of professional decision-making is useful to this study because it provides another means of understanding the dynamic assessment process that an assessor has to encompass in practice. In common with home treatment and the practice models (below), 'professional boundaries' have at their core the coming together of different professional frameworks (Goffman 1974), while at the same time they suggest the need for a broader framework within which to understand the assessment process.

Practice models

The use of models in terms of MHA assessments in the UK has been under-researched (Dunn 2001). An early example of such a model within the mental health literature of the early 1990s refers to social risk orientation (Sheppard 1990). By the early 2000s, a number of other models had been proposed and investigated in light of pending changes to the 1983 MHA and a growing interest in home treatment (Bridgett & Polak 2003; Peay 2003; Quirk et al. 2003), incorporating not only the notion of risk but also mental health team dynamics and the patient's social network. Nevertheless, there has been little progress in the conceptualisation of models of MHA assessments, despite the significant rise in the number of such assessments in the UK (Dunn 2001). Bridgett and Polak (2003) and (Johnson et al., 2004, 2005; Johnson & Needle 2008) have explored in some detail models of home treatment, but their findings refer to *all* people diverted from mental health hospital admissions, rather than just those solely assessed under the MHA (CQC 2015).

The social risk orientation model: *utilising a clinical approach*

Sheppard argues that key to understanding the ASW's role is a clear understanding of the MHA criteria of 'health and safety of the patient [and] protection of other people' (1990, p.vi). His model of good practice uses a Compulsory Admissions Assessment Framework, in the form of an ASW assessment audit schedule covering six classifications: hazards, mental health threat, physical ill-health threat, safety threat, protection of other people, and availability and adequacy of support (Sheppard 1993). Each classification has a number of questions rating the level of risk and danger, which are summarised at the end of the schedule so as to gain an overall rating of the risk. Glover and Johnson (2008); Glover–Thomas (2011) add to this assessment approach, although using the term 'Risk Recipe' model. Glover-Thomas draws on tort law, in which it is argued that a number of conditions come together to form a particular outcome. Using Sheppard's example, a combination of the six classifications would inform and guide the professional's assessment outcome. While the ASWs in principle found this model useful, they argue that there are many factors which could be combined and these combinations would produce an exhaustive list, hence while the Risk Recipe model is a valuable tool, it is not the sole arbiter to the decision-making process.

The team support model: *utilising a non-clinical approach*

The research of Quirk et al. (2003) on MHA assessments used a participant observation and interview data collection methodology which included direct observations of MHA assessments by five teams working in inner and outer London. Their study identified that a number of non-clinical and extra-legal influences had an effect on compulsory admissions to hospital. The non-clinical influences included insufficient time to set up alternatives to hospital admissions and being unsupported by other professionals. The extra-legal influences included structural operational norms and professional accountability of MHA decision-making at the agency level.

The social systems model: *utilising both a clinical and non-clinical approach*

The social systems approach (Bridgett & Polak 2003; Bridgett & Gijsman 2008) uses the principles of crisis intervention based on the early work of Caplan (1964). This model of crisis intervention not only considers the individual service user, but also incorporates the individual's social context as key to understanding their crisis. The model looks at how equilibrium can be re-established in a person's life and what has caused the disturbance to the person's social network. The model emphasises the positive opportunities that can be achieved in a crisis situation, due to an individual and their social system being more accepting of help at times of crisis. The principles of the model include ensuring coordination, adopting a social focus, encouraging communication and enabling coping.

Methodology

The study used an interpretive approach (Conrad and Barker 2010) informed by the work of Charmaz (2006). The research was undertaken within a large Mental Health Trust in the East of England, which served primarily an urban population. The purposive sample included all MHA assessments with an outcome of home treatment undertaken between January and March 2008. The Trust identified a total of 54 cases, of which nine cases were noted as having ASWs requesting home treatment as an outcome. The service users, ASWs and Home Treatment Professionals (HTPs) from the nine home treatment cases formed the sample group to be interviewed. Semi-structured interviewing was used so as to provide a systematic method of data collection from the ASWs' and HTPs' practice. All the interviews were audio-recorded and transcribed. Framework analysis was the method used to evaluate the qualitative data in a systematic way (Ritchie & Spencer 1994). Ethical approval for the research was sought and obtained from the NHS, National Research Ethics Service, England (08/H0302/76).

Findings: undertaking mental health act assessments

In the interviews conducted with the ASWs and HTPs undertaking MHA assessments, it was observed how their experiences 'fit' the conceptual frameworks described above (social crisis, negotiation and practice models), as assessors navigating their way through the assessment process. For the purpose of this article, three of the most significant themes have been selected, namely: mental illness or social crisis, negotiation and mental illness, and mental illness and social networks.

Mental illness or social crisis?

How ASWs and HTPs interpret both service users' behaviour and events permits a closer analysis of professional practice behaviour. Framing service users' behaviour and then acting on that understanding significantly influences how ASWs and HTPs practise and consequently what service provision is provided.

The social constructions of service users' worlds, as presented by the ASWs and HTPs, were notably different. The ASWs predominately explored service users' worlds and their problems in terms of social crises, while the HTPs identified service users' problems in terms of individual pathologies and risk. The ASWs explored, in some detail, the complex relationships and coping mechanisms utilised by service users in their attempts to resolve difficulties. ASW Adam[1] put words to this when explaining his understanding of one service user:

> …her drug taking, her psychotic behaviour and her quest for independence and rebellious behaviour was somewhat linked to this rather enmeshed family dynamic and they were basically treating her as if she was about 11 years old and so the

mother and father hadn't really begun this sort of natural disengagement process that you should do with a young adult. So they were being very, being over-parental. (ASW, case 7)

In addition, the ASWs pointed to causal relationships between social problems and a service user's mental health; for example, the breakdown of a close personal relationship which he/she is unable to come to terms with and their changing social status. The types of narrative varied within this social discourse, but included how the behaviour could be seen as a normal response to their social situation (i.e., finding it difficult to accept rejection by their partner and taking drastic measures to maintain contact with that person). ASW Andy, for example, identified in case 1 that a drug overdose had followed a break-up with the service user's boyfriend.

However, for the HTPs, the primary interest was the identification of a mental illness rather than gaining an understanding of the social context in which the service user presented. This can best be illustrated with regard to case 2, in which ASW Alan explored the complex social relationship of the service, but the HTP's initial intervention in this case focused on identifying a mental illness, the level of risk and looking for a diagnosis, then for a treatment for the diagnosis, with the social aspect of the problem being seen as secondary.

For the HTPs, clearly labelling a service user as having a mental illness was seen as a priority. Attempts to resolve this problem were undertaken by trying to classify service users into two groups ('mentally ill' and 'other') and being guarded as to who they selected as being 'mentally ill'. Analyses of the HTPs' narratives were therefore characterised by frequent references to the service users' mental disorders and the risks associated with those disorders.

The issue of trying to identify whether a service user is presenting with a social crisis or a mental illness is further complicated when this is their first presentation to the psychiatric services. In such a case, HTPs cannot rely on any previous history or an earlier diagnosis, and ASWs may not be able to gain key information about the service user. Therefore, it is sometimes difficult to identify whether their problem is caused by emotional distress or an underlying mental health problem, and thus whether HTPs would accept the case or not.

The language used by ASWs and HTPs reflected their different understandings and approaches to service users and their problems. The ASWs expressed their concerns for service users using language which reflects their relationships and the social context, while the HTPs focused on exploring service users' diagnoses and the negative implications of having a mental illness. For example, regarding their use of language, two ASWs stated that 'She self-describes as a total drama queen, and she was' (ASW, case 7) and '…a young man who has been to university, who has had some difficulties before…' (ASW, case 9). In comparison, two HTPs stated that '…there is a history with this patient, bipolar affective disorder, psychotic depression, anxiety' (HTP, case 7) and 'More important about them accepting that they have got a mental health problem' (HTP, case 9).

Negotiation and mental illness: autonomy and authority

The negotiations between the ASWs and HTPs, as explored in terms of risk in the previous section, provided the ASWs with considerable challenges regarding their negotiations for home treatment, as well as thought-provoking reflections regarding the HTPs' beliefs. ASWs thus find themselves in the role of negotiator, deal-maker and decision-maker when engaging with service users.

The ASW's role of negotiator and deal-maker in exploring community provision with service users would normally include, as part of the deal, a consensus regarding the plan between the ASW and the service user. For service users wishing to return home, part of the plan would be that they would accept the involvement of a Home Treatment Team (HTT).

In addition to the use of home treatment, some ASWs also attempted to secure other commitments from service users, depending upon the circumstances of the case, including commitments from the service user not to repeat their previous high-risk behaviour.

ASWs, in pursing home treatment or securing commitments from service users, have no powers of enforcing these requests – only powers to detain under the MHA (with the agreement of two medical doctors) if the service user does not agree to these requests. ASWs also have no direct access to home treatment and must negotiate access to the service. Additionally, assessments with HTPs are problematic due to HTPs having only limited decision-making autonomy; decisions are normally made collectively by the HTT.

Therefore, for ASWs to successfully negotiate access to home treatment, they have to address a number of difficulties. They need to negotiate a common understanding of mental illness with the HTT, agree a timescale for team decision-making, adhere to the resources available to the HTT, and ensure that the team feels secure with the decision-making of that ASW.

Mental illness and social networks – shared roles

The relationship between direct support from the service user's social network and the provision of home treatment also showed that the treatment provided can be seen as a shared role. Initially, it was identified that home treatment seemed to only provide one key 'treatment': medication. However, when using a broader interpretation of 'treatment', it was seen that home treatment also provides a wider range of therapies which relate to the service user's milieu. This milieu includes the contribution of the service user's own social support network and it was found that there is a considerable overlap between the treatment provided by the HTT and that provided by the family. The milieu of definable therapies includes (1) emotional support and medication, (2) response to crisis and (3) practical support, as described in Table 1.

Treatments: medication and emotional support

The dominant treatment to which all the HTPs referred was medication and this was seen as essential in any treatment provided to a service user receiving a home treatment service. In addition, the HPTs provide a form of unstructured talking therapy rather than specific therapies such as psychotherapy or cognitive behavioural therapy. These talking therapies are used as an opportunity to monitor the service user's frame of mind.

TABLE 1 Roles of home treatment and a service user's family/social network

Support/provision	Treatments: emotional support and medication		Response to crisis	Practical support
Family/social network	Emotional support: interpersonal	Monitoring of medication	Available to alert mental health professionals	Accommodation Meal provision Being available
Home treatment	Emotional support: coping strategies Crisis planning	Monitoring of medication and providing medication	Urgent monitoring of risk	Accommodation Respite care – hospital Sleep, hygiene Being available

Response to crises – Joint working between the HTPs and the service user's social network was also identified as a way of monitoring the service user's behaviour, providing an early warning to the HTPs if the family feels the situation is becoming problematic. This approach seems to partly address three issues that the HPTs have: 24 h monitoring by the HTT is not possible, the family could supplement shortages when HTT staff are not available, and may provide additional information to the HTPs.

Practical support – While some types of practical support could be undertaken by HTPs or the close family (for example, shopping or meal provision), some practical support such as accessing accommodation for the homeless has to be negotiated by HTPs rather than family members. The HTPs look for the family to take on a supportive role. Non-clinical roles where possible are allocated to the family. It is also recognised that the HTPs not only work with the service users but also their family members.

Discussion

Limitations

This research was conducted in one Trust are only, using a small sample, so it is not possible to generalise what these findings would mean for the wider population of mental health social workers carrying out such statutory functions elsewhere. One of the greatest challenges in this research was gaining access to service user participants. After a six-month period of attempting to engage service users, it was recognised that engaging this sample group was not going to be practical. The problem of engaging service users was not unique to this study (Bailey & Liyange 2012).

An integrated assessment journey

The experience of assessors undertaking MHA assessments can be compared to a journey in which the destination at the start is unknown. However, Matthews, O'Hare, and Hemmington (2014); O'Hare (2014), in common with the majority of respondents in my study, found that this journey was undertaken within a climate in which assessors were required 'to make sense of a range of disparate and conflicting information, and abiding by complex law and Codes of Practice' (O'Hare 2014, p.173). For some research participants, there was a very real concern that the problems of the service user may be fundamentally more of a social nature than a medical one. Some of the ASWs explored the behaviour of the service users, whereby they considered in detail the context in which that behaviour took place. For HTPs, this exploration of social relationships was not seen as their primary role, it was about clarifying whether the person had a mental illness which could be quantified in terms of a diagnosis and risk. The ASWs and HTPs had both common and conflicting interests, whereby they engaged with each other to endeavour to reach a form of mutually beneficial service for the service user, while recognising that the other party does not always share their own values, interests, goals and ethical principles (Ferraro & Briody 2017).

It is significant to note that many of the participants recognise the complexity of the negotiation process, in which ASWs and HTPs need to reach a common ground to move forward. The relationship between ASWs and HTPs was seen as a key issue in gaining consensus. It should be noted that ASWs only have their powers of persuasion when asking HTPs to take a case - they have no power to enforce their requests. Failure to engage the HTP and team would, more than likely from the study findings, tip the balance in favour of hospital admission.

It should be noted that the participants in this study were only exploring cases in which alternatives to hospital admission were being pursued, and where the service users could have been detained under the MHA. This group of practitioners have been shown to be experienced, thoughtful, reflective and articulate about their practice. These individuals were able to draw upon a range of assessment experiences, considerable periods in practice and having worked in multiple team settings. The ASWs recognised that each assessment was a unique experience, in which they constantly questioned the decisions they made and recognised the complexity of the task, as well as the many options available to them. Thus, these ASWs operate in a way which closely resembles Peay's (2003) ethical decision-maker, while not ignoring other decision-makers' views. This is in sharp contrast to Gorovitz's (1982) observations, in which practitioners often assert that they wish that they could do something and then don't do it, when this preferred route of action is perfectly feasible.

The ASWs in this study gave a significantly high priority to home treatment outcomes, showing that they understood the complexity of the practice setting rather than the view suggested by Gorovitz that ASWs do not recognise that they can 'choose over a much wider range of options than [they] realize' (1982, p.68). For these ASWs, the sense of achievement in engaging HTPs did not outweigh other aspects; for example, the pragmatic nature of the ASWs' practice and the need to 'identify the present reality' rather than have preconceptions of mental illness and risk.

Thus, for the ASWs, the concern to clarify or gain a better understanding of the social crisis or mental illness was central to the debate. Nevertheless, the uncertainty associated with MHA assessments was seen to be ever-present in the accounts of the participants. The social crisis/social justice (Cahn 2000) approach that the ASWs took thus informed the type of data they gathered and hence their formulation of the assessment outcome.

Conclusion: implications for contemporary practice

In conclusion, then, what does the research have to say about contemporary mental health care practice for social workers who undertake the Approved Mental Health Practitioner role, in particular, in relation to providing the least restrictive outcome when assessing people under the MHA?

MHA assessments clearly cross the health and social care divide, and thus professional shared decision-making makes a significant impact on a service user's experience, affecting both their present and future. According to Fook:

> Because difference [narratives] is often constructed in a binary and oppositional manner, different categories may become fixed. And because they are often determined by the dominant discourse, then the different categories that are created often preserve dominant categorisations and hierarchies (Fook 2012, p.93)

It is this dominant medical narrative which has been critically explored in this study, so as to consider how alternative narratives can influence outcomes and, specifically, the use of home treatment as a community resource.

It could be argued that co-production (Cahn 2000) could offer a model in which professionals can work with other professionals, not only at the point of assessment but also beyond the assessment process, by seeing service users as assets who have a role to play during and beyond the assessment process. Understanding service users' social capital is paramount, whereby professionals, communities and families all understand the complex relationships involving a range of services, obligations and, especially, all gain a mutual understanding and exchange of what it means to have a significant life crisis.

My intention here has been to highlight the fact that the intricacies of MHA assessments and the models used are poorly understood in the UK and that decision-making during the assessment process may be characterised by uncertainty and negative risk taking. However, this research also considers how alternative constructions of MHA assessments can be envisaged, in which life-changing opportunities to support a person in crisis are explored. There are many lessons to be learnt; for example, about the way language is used and communicated and what support is appropriate to people being assessed under the MHA – but critically there needs to be a recognition that decisions made during the assessment process can have life-changing consequences for service users. Building on Hugman's (Hugman 1998, p.68) 'value choices', good practice in this area must be based on a wider consensus of what constitutes an MHA assessment. Social workers, who undertake the majority of MHA assessments, would seem to be well-placed to develop the concept of co-production within the assessment process, so as to help professionals and service users make sense of what is taking place during their crisis, and to assist professionals to recognise the complex narratives that inform their decision-making.

Note

1. All names anonymised.

References

Bailey, D., & Liyange, L. (2012). The role of the mental health social worker: political pawns in the reconfiguration of adult health and social care. *British Journal of Social Work, 42*, 1113–1131.

Barber, P., Brown, R., & Martin, D. (2012). *Mental health law in England and Wales: A guide for mental health professionals*. Exeter: Learning Matters.

Barnes, M. (1990). Assessing for compulsory detention: Applying the social perspective. *Research, Policy and Planning, 8*(1), 1–11.

Barnes, M., Bowl, R., & Fisher, M. (1990). *Sectioned: Social services and the 1983 mental health act*. London: Routledge.

Booth, T., Melotte, D., Philips, D., Pritlove, J., Barritt, A., & Lightup, R. (1985). Psychiatric crisis in the community: Collaboration and the 1983 mental health act. In G. Horobin (Ed.), *Responding to mental illness* (pp. 71–88). New York, NY: St. Martin's Press.

Bowl, R., Barnes, M., & Fisher, M. (1987). A real alternative. *Community Care*, 26–28.

Bridgett, C., & Gijsman, H. (2008). Working with families and social networks. In S. Johnson, J. Needle, & G. Thornicroft (Eds.), *Crisis resolution and home treatment in mental health* (pp. 177–195). Cambridge: Cambridge University Press.

Bridgett, C., & Polak, P. (2003). Social systems intervention and crisis resolution: Part 1: Assessment. *Advances in Psychiatric Treatment, 9*, 424–431.

Cahn, E. (2000). *No more throw-away people: The co-production imperative*. Washington, DC: Essential; Charlbury: Jon Carpenter [distributor].

Campbell, J. (2010). Deciding to detain: The use of compulsory mental health law by UK. *British Journal of Social Work, 40*(1), 328–334.

Caplan, G. (1964). *Principles of preventative psychiatry*. London: The Tavistock Institute.

Charmaz, K. (2006). *Constructing grounded theory: A practical guide through qualitative analysis*. London: Sage.

Conrad, P, & Barker, K. (2010). The Social Construction of Illness: Key Insights and Policy Implications. *Journal of Health and Social Behaviour, 51* (S), s67–s79.

Coppock, V., & Dunn, B. (2010). *Understanding social work practice in mental health*. Los Angeles, CA: Sage.

CQC (2014). *Monitoring the mental health act in 2012/13*. London: CQC.

CQC (2015). *Monitoring the mental health act in 2015/16*. London: CQC.

Davidson, G, & Campbell, J. (2010). An audit of assessment and recording by approved social workers (ASWs). *British Journal of Social Work, 40*, 1609–1627.

DoH (1999). *A national service framework for mental health: Modern standards and service models*. London: DoH.

DoH (2001). *The mental health policy implementation guide*. London: DoH.

Dunn, L. (2001). Mental health act assessments: Does a community treatment team make a difference? *International Journal of Social Psychiatry, 47*, 1–19.

Ferraro, G., & Briody, E. (2017). *The cultural dimension of global business* (8th ed.). London: Taylor & Francis.

Fisher, M., Barnes, M., & Bowl, R. (1987). Monitoring the mental health act 1983: Implications for policy and practice. *Research, Policy and Planning, 5*, 1–8.

Fook, J. (2012). *Social work: A critical approach to practice*. London: Sage.

Glover, G., & Johnson, S. (2008). The crisis resolution team model: Recent developments and dissemination. In S. Johnson, J. Needle, & G. Thornicroft (Eds.), *Crisis resolution and home treatment in mental health* (pp. 117–176). Cambridge: Cambridge University Press.

Glover-Thomas, N. (2011). The age of risk: Risk perception and determination following the mental health act 2007. *Medical Law Review, 19*, 25.

Goffman, E. (1974). *Frame analysis: An essay on the organization of experience*. London: Penguin Books.

Golightley, M. (2014). *Social work and mental health*. Exeter: Learning Matters.

Gorovitz, S. (1982). *Doctors' dilemmas: Moral conflict and medical care*. Oxford: Oxford University Press.

Gregor, C. (2010). Unconscious aspects of statuary mental health social work: Emotional labour and the approved mental health professional. *Journal of Social Work Practice, 24*(4), 429–443.

Hall, P. (1995). *A comparison of two social service departments' introduction of the purchaser/provider separation and the effects on their mental health teams* (Unpublished Masters Dissertation). London: Brunel University.

Hall, P. (2015). *An examination of mental health act assessments and the use of home treatment* (Unpublished Doctoral Thesis). Essex: University of Essex.

Hugman, R. (1998). *Social Welfare and Social Value*. London: Macmillan.

Huntington, J. (1981). *Social work and medical practice: Collaboration or conflict?*. London: George Allen and Unwin.

Johnson, S. (2004). Crisis resolution and intensive home treatment teams. *Community Psychiatry, 1*, 22–25.

Johnson, S., & Needle, J. (2008). Crisis resolution teams: Rational and core model. In S. Johnson, J. Needle, J. P. Bindman, & G. Thornicroft (Eds.), *Crisis resolution and home treatment in mental health* (pp. 67–84). Cambridge: Cambridge University Press.

Johnson, S., Bingham, C., Billings, J., Pilling, S., Morant, N., Bebbington, P. E., … Dalton, J. (2004). Woman's experiences of admission to a crisis house and to a acute hospital wards: A qualitative study. *Journal of Mental Health, 13*, 247–262.

Johnson, S., Nolan, P. S., Pilling, S., Sandor, A., Hoult, J., McKenzie, N., … Bebbington, P. (2005). Randomised controlled trial of acute mental health care by a crisis resolution team: The North Islington crisis study. *British Medical Journal, 331*, 1–5.

Kinney, M. (2010). Being assessed under the 1983 mental health act – Can it ever be ethical? *Ethics and Social Welfare, 3*(3), 329–336.

Langan, J. (1989). *Factors approved social workers take into account when using the compulsory powers under the mental health act 1983* (Unpublished M.Sc. dissertation). Department of Social Work, University of East Anglia, Norwich.

Matthews, S., O'Hare, P., & Hemmington, J. (2014). *Approved mental health practice: Essential themes for students and practitioners*. Basingstoke: Palgrave Macmillan.

O'Hare, P. (2014). Evidence-based practice. In P. O'Hare (Ed.), *Approved mental health practice: Essential themes for students and practitioners* (pp. 171–186). Basingstoke: Palgrave Macmillan.

Peay, J. (2003). *Decisions and dilemmas: Working with mental health law*. Oxford: Hart.

Quirk, A., Lelliott, P., Audini, B., & Buston, K. (2003). Non-clinical and extra-legal influences on decisions about compulsory admission to psychiatric hospital. *Journal of Mental Health, 12*, 119–130.

Ritchie, J., & Spencer, L. (1994). Qualitative data analysis for applied policy research. In A. Bryman & R. G. Burgess (Eds.), *Analyzing qualitative data* (pp. 173–194). London: Routledge.

Schon, D. (1987). *Educating the reflective practitioner*. San Francisco, CA: Jossey-Bass.

Sheppard, M. (1990). *Mental health: The role of the approved social worker*. Sheffield: Joint Unit for Social Services Research, Sheffield University in collaboration with Community Care Journal.

Sheppard, M. (1993). Theory for approval social work: The use of the compulsory admissions assessment schedule. *British Journal of Social Work, 23*, 231–257.

Tew, J. (2005). *Social perspectives in mental health: Developing social models to understand and work with mental distress*. London: Jessica Kingsley.

Jane Fenton and Timothy B. Kelly

'RISK IS KING AND NEEDS TO TAKE A BACKSEAT!' CAN SOCIAL WORKERS' EXPERIENCES OF MORAL INJURY STRENGTHEN PRACTICE?

This paper considers the idea that moral injury may result from social workers being exposed to sustained ethical stress – the stress experienced when workers cannot base their practice on their values. It is suggested that a particularly salient feature of agency working which might contribute to the experience of ethical stress is risk aversion. This paper is based on a study of one hundred criminal justice social workers in Scotland, who were questioned on their experiences of ethical stress and risk aversion. Quantitative and qualitative data were collected and analysed using standard multiple regression and inductive thematic analysis, respectively. Findings demonstrated that how risk-averse an agency was contributed in a unique and significant way to the worker's experience of ethical stress. Qualitative comments illustrated why this relationship might exist, but also demonstrated that a variety of views were held by social workers and that ethical stress was not experienced by all. The findings are discussed in terms of moral injury and its links with risk aversion, bureaucracy, neoliberal hegemony, notions of 'underclass', personal moral codes and professional integrity. Explicitly exploring these related concepts in social work education might impact on the new generation of social workers and strengthen the profession.

Introduction

Moral injury initially referred to shame and guilt disturbances experienced by combat veterans and it manifested in some of the symptoms of posttraumatic stress disorder (Frankfurt & Frazier 2016). In recent years, the concept has gained traction and there is a small but growing body of literature and research about moral injury, almost exclusively relating to the atrocities of war. A widely accepted definition of moral injury is put forward by Litz et al. (2009) and Drescher et al. (2011, p.9). They suggest that moral injury is a *disruption in an individual's confidence and expectations about one's own or others' motivation or capacity to behave in a just and ethical manner. This injury is brought about by bearing witness to perceived immoral acts, failure to stop such actions, or perpetration of immoral acts, in particular actions that are inhumane, cruel, depraved or violent, bringing about pain, suffering, or death of others.* Boudreau (2011), writing from his own personal experience as a war veteran says that moral injury describes the wounds a person inflicts on him/herself when he or she inflicts wounds on another. It is the damage that is done to one's own moral fibre when one does the transgressing. When a person accepts these transgressions – a piece of his/her moral integrity is sacrificed, and this is the essence of moral injury.

Litz and his colleagues (2009) postulate a process model of moral injury. They suggest that the process begins with the experience of a transgression. This experience creates a dissonance or conflict in ones sense of self. If a person is unable to assimilate the experience into existing cognitive schemas of one's sense of self then shame, guilt and anxiety occur. This leads to withdrawal and a failure to forgive one's self and feelings of self-condemnation. Finally, the person will experience chronic thought intrusions, avoidance, numbing, self-harming, self-handicapping and demoralisation.

There is some tautological and conceptual confusion in the literature around moral injury. Some suggest that moral injury occurs when one experiences morally injurious events. For example, Shay (2014) says moral injury 'is present when 1) there has been a betrayal of what's right 2) by someone who holds legitimate authority 3) in a high stakes situation' (p.183). Blinka and Harris (2016) also conflate process and outcome. Frankfurt and Frazier (2016) helpfully separate transgressive acts from the outcomes of experiencing transgressive acts. They use Litz and colleagues' (2009) understanding of morally injurious behaviours as a definition of transgressive acts. Namely, transgressive acts are 'perpetrating, failing to prevent, bearing witness to, or learning about acts that transgress deeply help moral beliefs and expectations' (Litz et al. 2009, p.700). Moral injury is one potential outcome of experiencing transgressive acts. This differentiation is consistent with the model proposed by Litz and colleagues (2009).

As indicated earlier, most of the literature and research pertaining to moral injury is related to extreme experiences in war or military occupations. We believe that the concept of moral injury may be applicable to experiences that are not as extreme or potentially acutely traumatising as experiences in war. In drawing on these concepts we wish to make it explicitly clear that we are not likening the experiences of professional social work practice to the horrors and traumatic events that soldiers may experience whether within or outwith the wartime rules of engagement. However, we do believe that practice in many professions can expose professionals to situations where they may experience transgressive acts, acts that go against deeply help personal or professional values. This exposure to transgressive acts may lead to the development of moral injury, albeit of a lesser order than that which is experienced in contexts of war.

We are beginning to see this non-military application of moral injury reflected in a few recent publications (e.g. Levinson 2015 – teacher education; Reamer 2014 – social work; Woods 2016 – undercover policing). Take, for example, Finefter-Rosenbluh's (2016) explorations of teachers' experiences of moral injury when engaging in reflective activities required, and mandated, for a professional development programme. The procedural format of the programme comprised quite rigid rules to be followed and Finefter-Rosehbluh found that the study participants reported strong feelings of discomfort when they were unable to do what felt 'right' due to the restrictions of the procedures. The author concludes that the teachers were suffering moral injury as a result of having to follow restrictive procedures when they felt the action was wrong. Di Franks (2008) found that when social workers had to practice in a managerial and gatekeeping manner that was not congruent with their values, they suffered high levels what he termed 'disjuncture'. Fenton's work (2014a) extends the idea of disjuncture to include ontological guilt (the feeling experienced when a person feels they cannot act in accordance with their conscience) (Taylor 2007), bringing both concepts together in a notion of 'ethical stress'.

It may be that ethical stress is a lower level of moral injury. Litz's and colleagues' (2009) process model of moral injury begins with the experience of transgressive acts. A social worker may find ways to overlook or excuse such transgression, leading to what Boudreau (2011) describes as sacrifice of a piece of one's moral integrity. We argue that such sacrifices may move beyond ethical stress and cause moral injury, especially if workers are exposed to transgressive acts over a prolonged period of time.

Thus far, then, it is suggested that moral injury can result from sustained managerial, formulaic and procedural expectations that constrain or inhibit value-based, responsive practice. It has also been reported widely in the literature that risk preoccupation in social work is a powerful manifestation of managerialism, based on the neoliberal idea of managing the behaviour of risky people (Rogowski 2015). Couple this to neoliberal ideas of service users as architects of their own misfortune, and the social work task becomes one of risk assessment and correcting individual behaviour. Any ethical impulse towards helping or building a relationship is undermined in this context.

Also, as Webb (2006) states, 'social work has sunk into a 'managerialism' that is increasingly afraid of the complexity of risk decisions and has become highly defensive' (Webb 2006, p.1). In other words, social work is afraid of complex risk decisions in case things go wrong, and therefore practice *defensively* in order to show that they have 'done things right' (as opposed to having 'done the right things) (Munro 2011, p.6). Such defensive organisational cultures appear to negatively impact on early career workers (Chenot, Benton, & Kim 2009) as well as more experienced workers (Jones 2001; Preston-Shoot 2003).

Given the above, then, it might be suggested that restrictive, procedural and risk-averse practice contexts would be environments where moral injury might burgeon. We now turn to an empirical study which explores this connection.

Methodology

This paper is drawn from the findings of a wider research project conducted across four criminal justice departments in four separate local authority areas in Scotland (Fenton 2014a). The four local authorities were conveniently sampled from a possible 32 to provide a contrast between rural and urban areas and to provide enough participants for the study, whilst not creating untenable demands on the researcher's available time and resources. The authors had no previous employment with any of the four local authorities.

Using a within-stage mixed-model study design (Johnson & Onwuegbuzie, 2004), the relationships between the experience of ethical stress and agency variables were explored. The agency variables, drawn from a review of the literature, were 'how we work with offenders', 'agency approach to risk' and 'ethical climate of the agency'.

The research was operationalised via questionnaires designed to elicit both quantitative and qualitative data. Two hundred and forty questionnaires were distributed to all basic-grade criminal justice social workers in the four local authorities and 100 usable questionnaires were returned, which is a response rate of 42%.

The questionnaire was designed in sections, each section concerned with measuring one of the variables. Likert-style questions were utilised to elicit the quantitative data, and each section ended with an opportunity for respondents to make comment as they wished. In this paper, we are concerned with the variable 'agency approach to risk' and its relationship with ethical stress.

Ethical approval for the study was obtained from the authors' institutional ethics committee and from each local authority.

Validity

Validity is the strength of any tool or questionnaire in measuring what it sets out to measure (Fischer & Corcoran 2007). The first step in investigating the validity of the questionnaire was to undertake a 'logical content analysis' (Fischer & Corcoran 2007, p.125), which is the explicit demonstration of the literature basis of each question in the questionnaire. For example, sample questions pertaining to the risk variable and the ethical stress measure were shown in Table 1.

Post data collection, a test of 'convergent validity' was undertaken which is a measure of how 'scores on a measure converge with theoretically relevant variables' (Fischer & Corcoran 2007, p.14). The correlation between ethical stress measures and the other variables was therefore investigated using Pearson product–moment correlation coefficient. The resultant score for the relationship between the risk variable and ethical stress was .717, which is considered a 'large' correlation (Pallant 2010, p.134). From this, we can infer that those sections of the questionnaire had robust convergent validity.

The questionnaire was piloted with a group of nine social work academics and practising social workers and amendments made as suggested.

Reliability

According to Rudestam and Newton (2007), it is essential to ensure that any questionnaire is reliable, which can be ascertained by measuring internal consistency; a measure of whether the items in each of the questionnaire variable subscales are tapping into

TABLE 1 Sample logical content analysis

Variable	Question	Literature basis
Agency approach to risk	'Risk-averse' describes my agency well	Kemshall (2002), Webb (2006), Phillips (2009), Taylor (2007), Barry (2007)
Ethical stress	I experience stress because I am not always able to help my clients in the way I want to	Kosny and Eakin (2008), Jones (2001), Preston-Shoot (2003), Fenton (2012)
Ethical Stress	When I have to follow procedures that don't feel 'right' it causes stress	Taylor (2007)

the same phenomenon. A Cronbach's coefficient alpha of .8 or above for a subscale is, according to Fischer and Corcoran (2007), a measure of good internal consistency. 'Agency approach to risk', and 'ethical stress' scales produced Cronbach's coefficient alpha of .872 and .817, respectively, demonstrating good internal consistency.

Analysis

Analysis of the quantitative data was carried out using SPSS (2007) for Windows, version 16.0. A standard multiple regression was undertaken between the three combined variables ('agency approach to risk', 'how we work with offenders' and 'ethical climate of the agency') and the experience of ethical stress, and results demonstrated that the combined variables contributed significantly to the experience of ethical stress. Beta values of the variables were then checked to ascertain which were contributing to the result.

In relation to the qualitative data, an inductive thematic analysis (Carey 2009) was carried out on the 80 free text comments by the primary author. The process involved identifying initial themes, categorisation of the themes, followed by a refinement of the themes and sub-themes. The second author independently performed an audit of the theme development, checking the links between text and final themes.

Results

According to the results from the standard multiple regression, the perception of the 'agency approach to risk' was found to make a unique and significant contribution to the experience of ethical stress.

The statistical relationship between 'agency approach to risk' and ethical stress:

	Beta value	Significance
Agency approach to risk	.341	.009 ($p < .01$)

In essence, the scale measured how risk-averse the respondent viewed their agency, and there was a significant finding that that the more risk-averse the agency is perceived to be, the more ethical stress or moral injury is experienced by the social worker. This variable had the strongest effect on the experience of ethical stress.

In terms of the qualitative data, there were 80 free text comments and most concerned risk, either directly or as an associated issue. Examples of comments dealing directly with risk were:

Risk is king and needs to take a back seat!

There is a major emphasis on risk assessment.

We constantly hear about defensible decisions

Public protection is seen as our utmost aim

Discussion

Limitations

The central limitation of the study is that it was located within a very particular social work context – criminal justice services in Scotland. However, work with people who have offended in Scotland is part of the social work department and is bound by the same legislation, that is, the Social Work (Scotland) Act 1968, with its central tenet of promoting social welfare. The work is also framed by the Scottish Social services Council's Code of Practice (SSSC 2016), British Association of Social Work's code of ethics (British Association of Social Workers [BASW] 2012) and the International Federation of Social Workers' standards of practice (IFSW 2012). Findings also resonate with much of the literature on risk aversion pertaining to social work more widely so generalisation may be possible. Also, only four local authority areas were studied and perhaps a different picture would have emerged had all local authority CJSW departments in Scotland been examined.

There were also some limitations in terms of study methods in that the questionnaire was lengthy and might have deterred busy social workers from participating in the study. Also, had time allowed for follow-up focus groups or interviews, rather than the reliance on free-text comments, a deeper interpretation of the data might have been possible.

Connections to risk aversion

The quantitative finding implies that social workers experience significant ethical stress when risk aversion stifles value-based practice. This would suggest that social workers, in the main, view values as important and central to practice but that rigid, risk-averse contexts can inhibit their application. Analysis of the free text comments pertaining to risk can help illuminate why this might be. Comments were identified as having a relationship with two sub-themes: bureaucracy; and neoliberal ideas of 'underclass'.

Moral injury from risk aversion and bureaucracy

Broadhurst, Hall, Wastell, White, and Pithouse (2010) describe an ideological commitment to the technical–rational implementation of risk assessment and management processes in children's services, which unavoidably, and intentionally, involves instruments, procedures, tools, forms and structured formats; in other words, bureaucracy. The authors discuss the seductive potential of these technologies as leading to certainty and ensuring no mistakes are made. Littlechild (2010, p.668) calls this the 'actuarial fallacy' as, of course risk decisions can never be 'certain'. Munro (2011) in her review of child protection was also cautionary in regards to trying to achieve certainty, and explicitly condemned the over-bureaucratisation of children's services. It can be considered, therefore, that one manifestation of risk aversion that might well contribute to moral injury is bureaucracy. For example, one social worker in the study commented:

> I am in a very bureaucratic environment where engagement (with offenders) is viewed very disdainfully

For the social worker who made this comment, the erosion of engagement led them to feel heightened ethical stress or moral injury.

Bauman (2000, p.9) states: 'when we obscure the essential human and moral aspects of care behind even more rules and regulations, we make the daily practice of social work even more distant from its original ethical impulse'. Risk assessment, and risk-averse procedures rely heavily on bureaucracy – doing things correctly to demonstrate that diligence has been shown and that the agency cannot be open to criticism. This leads to a preoccupation with the bureaucratic elements of practice, often at the expense of actual social work with people. Bauman (1989, p.15) notes 'how formal and ethically blind is the bureaucratic pursuit of efficiency'. Another social worker stated:

> When I first came into social work, we were encouraged to look at the whole person ... more recent years have seen a major emphasis on risk instead and we are all about achieving targets

Bauman, of course, is very well known for his work on the Holocaust – and especially the distancing effects of bureaucracy. Overwhelming bureaucracy led to emotional and cognitive distance between decision-makers and the horrendous consequences. In essence, Bauman draws on Arendt's phrase to suggest that bureaucracy removes decision-makers from the 'animal pity' that it is part of the human condition to experience (Ardent 1964 in Bauman 1989, p.20). The 'animal pity' is the emotional and visceral reaction that one human usually has when faced with another human in distress. Bauman discusses how the modern inclination to break processes down into discreet tasks means that people become only interested in the completion of their task well, and feel dissociated from the eventual, actual outcome. Such disassociation from emotion is problematic as it makes social work practice inhumane (Taylor 2017).

Smith (2011) suggests that this technical–rational bureaucratic managerialism, has seduced social work into believing that the very complex and human problems it deals with can have reductionist, procedural and regulatory solutions. Evidence that it is *not* working, however, is often then absorbed into a redefinition of the task, which becomes the management of groups of risky people without the attempt to effect change. Technical–rational checklists, risk assessments, risk management plans and all manner of other procedures, then, are successful in surveillance, managing and reporting *and* in making sure the agency is safe from blame – 'the task is managerial, not transformative' (Feeley & Simon 1992, p.452).

The last point above illustrates a social work practice where moral injury would not result. Workers might feel happy that they are doing a good job in the task-focused manner explored by Bauman, and managers, concerned with audits and paperwork might reinforce this. This would be especially true when dealing with matters of risk. For example:

> I feel that social workers can be easily blamed if something goes wrong, so it is important to defend our practice.

The worker quoted above is one of a group who have no difficulty with the increasingly technical and bureaucratic approach to social work as the priority task is understood as keeping themselves safe from blame. The phrase 'if something goes wrong' identifies this comment as perhaps being influenced by a defensive, risk-averse attitude.

However, *if* social workers have a concern with really trying to help people, to affect change and to work in partnership with service users, then they may well feel morally and ethically compromised. Getting close to people, building a relationship and practising in a value-based way is very likely to provide the impetus towards 'animal pity' or, put in a less dramatic way, compassion and care for the people we are working with. What happens to those feelings when the social worker is not 'allowed' to be properly responsive – to take risks, to help and to get alongside service users? The current study and other authors (for example, Jones 2001; Preston-Shoot 2003) would suggest that, in those circumstances, social workers do become disillusioned and unhappy. This situation can also mean that a positive view of risk-taking as outlined by authors such as Taylor (2017) and Carson and Bain (2008), is eroded, frowned upon or simply not allowed. We would suggest that social workers in this context are experiencing moral injury as their ethical and helping impulses and degraded within restrictive and distant bureaucracies.

The technical, procedural work involved with risk assessment and management is an acute example of the above distancing nature of bureaucracy and workers' feelings about it can be seen in some of their comments:

> During weeks when there seems to be lots of deadlines, it can be stressful and you feel like you are letting clients down

> Modern social work practice is increasingly shifting focus to 'box-ticking' and 'number-crunching.' Lots of time is now spent on recording events.
> There is a major emphasis on risk assessment

> We are hamstrung by the plethora of forms we are required to complete. We spend 80% of our time inputting data into the various IT interfaces we have to utilise to maintain records, to undertake formal risk assessments and to record key performance indicators in order that our funding can be justified/secured. Work becomes more risk led – with 'resources following risk' at the expense of valuable preventative work for those offenders at the lower end of the scale.

It can be seen, then, that risk aversion is intrinsically linked to bureaucracy. If the emphasis is on prioritising the safety of the agency as opposed to doing the right thing in terms of being responsive to service users, then documentation and procedure are the most important elements of the practice. Comments above suggest that that is indeed the context of the agencies in the study and, unsurprisingly, some social workers feel moral injury when they cannot respond in the way they want to.

Moral injury from risk aversion and the neoliberal 'underclass' hegemony

Another aspect of risk aversion is its congruence with underpinning neoliberal ideology. In discussion of the 'culture' of agencies, Schein (2010, p.27) suggests that 'basic underlying assumptions' colour the culture of an agency, regardless of espoused values. If the basic underlying assumptions are informed by neoliberal hegemony then the idea of a social work service user as an individual completely responsible for their own misfortunes and simply requiring to correct their thinking and behaviour, fits very neatly. This construct of a service user fits very well with broader ideas around 'underclass:' a concept which has gained significant traction in the public's imagination in recent years (Jones 2011).

'Underclass' is a notion highlighted by Murray (1990), an American sociologist, who suggested that there is an 'underclass' in the United Kingdom, comprised of un-employed, criminal people who neglect their children and whose behaviour is the main contributory factor to the raft of social problems experienced by some communities. This idea is challenged by authors such as Jones (2011) whose thesis considers how the 'underclass' can become situated within the public imagination through clever manipula-tion by the media, by politicians and by the establishment whose ends are served by per-petuating the idea that people are poor or in difficult circumstances through their own fecklessness, not as a result a societal disadvantage and oppression. This is, of course, in keeping with neoliberal ideology where 'poor people, so the neoliberal view goes, remain poor as a result of bad choices and problematic behaviour' (Turbett 2014, p.12).

Fenton (2014b) demonstrated that younger, newer social workers were happier with hegemony-informed managerial, neoliberal social work practice and Gilligan (2007) found that the age group of students termed by the author as 'Thatcher's Chil-dren' were significantly more likely to define societal problems as the 'fault' of individ-ual behaviour and poor choices, rather than as arising from wider societal problems. It is also the case that society's attitudes to poor people, for example, have hardened over the preceding decades (Joseph Rowntree Foundation 2014). Many younger, newer workers and students, who have been steeped in over 30 years of neoliberalism, appear to have internalised the associated underpinning ethical assumptions of neoliberalism. Once these neoliberal ideas of an 'underclass' have taken hold then the social work task *does* morph into managing people and coercing them into changing their behaviour re-gardless of, or without taking cognisance of, the real barriers to change that might im-pact – poverty and inequality, for example. In this world, ethical stress or moral injury is very unlikely to be experienced because workers feel justified in authoritarian, man-agerial and distant practice. So, for example, some of the respondents to the study said:

The stress in the job is more about resistant clients and managing the risk they pose

This (offending) is through their choice

The comments above, then, demonstrate that there is a neoliberal framing of social work by some workers that is congruent with the idea that there is an underclass group who just need to make better choices and change their behaviour. Notions of care, compassion, understanding and help need not feature. Moral injury, again, would not result for those workers.

Once again, then, when social workers *do* want to engage properly with people, they might find themselves thwarted not only by heavy bureaucracy, risk aversion and managerial practice, but also by the prevailing, neoliberal attitudes of some workers and by the underpinning basic assumptions of the agency:

Engagement with services users is viewed very disdainfully

I don't think within the team I work that there is a sense that humanising what we do is relevant

Those workers who understand social problems in a wider, critical sense as more complex than simply bad behaviour know that people have potential and good qualities that circumstances do not allow to thrive. Hennessey (2011) discusses the importance of social workers engaging with services users' 'inner worlds' as well as their 'outer worlds'. The 'inner world' consists of the person's thoughts, feelings, understanding, sense making, aspirations, etc. Neoliberal social workers may not see the necessity in engaging with service users in that way, which might be a reason why service users often say they are not listened to, whilst highlighting that being listened to is one of the most important features of the social work relationship. As Beresford (2012) states:

> Service users frequently report how much they value social workers 'listening' to them. This quality or skill of being able to listen is the basis for much else that service users value. It makes them feel that they are valued, that their viewpoint has merit. It is the starting point for an approach to practice based on 'co-production' – the social worker working with the service user to find out what will help – the basis for all good practice.

Instead, if workers concentrate on services users' 'outer worlds' that is, their behaviour, then preoccupation with the 'visible' – risk factors, past misdemeanours, parents not attending appointments, not getting the children up for school, for example – can supplant any attempts to engage in what is going on in the service user's 'inner world'. Herein lies the clear link between 'underclass' thinking and risk aversion – to properly document risk factors and complete risk assessments, the focus has to be on behaviour and objective measurement and observation. Relationship-based, caring practice need not feature.

So, if social workers want to engage with service users and their 'inner worlds', the distancing effects of neoliberal 'underclass' thinking and the prioritisation of technical–rational risk assessment and management can lead to moral injury.

> Pressure is on to risk assess everyone, at the expense of getting to know, and work with, clients

> Conscience pricks me when have to do lengthy admin tasks when time could be better spent working with people

Moral injury, moral health, moral courage and risk

It is clear from the exploration in this paper so far that not all social workers will experience moral injury. There is a group of social workers and students who do not find that managerial and bureaucratic imperatives and the erosion of relationship based, caring social work cause them any kind of ethical stress or moral injury. In fact some of those social workers actively embrace the emphasis on risk assessment bureaucracy:

> I think it's a positive change in practice that work is based upon structured risk assessment tools

> Structured risk assessment tools only add to the professionalism of my work, by giving a sound research base on which to base decisions

Does this mean that those workers are, therefore, uninjured and, thus, more morally healthy? From the exploration of the ideas so far, it would seem that moral health is *not* implied by lack of moral injury. In fact, moral injury would affect those workers and students who have a very robust value base and a strongly held commitment to ethics and social justice. Given that the value base of social work is so concerned with social justice (for example, BASW Code of Ethics and the IFSW definition of social work), it might be suggested that only those workers who have professional and moral integrity might experience moral injury. Moral injury, therefore, might indeed be an impetus for good.

Supporting the above suggestion, Weinberg (2016) found that the personal discourse used by a social worker influenced how they viewed a social work dilemma or paradox. The social workers worked with young mothers at risk of having their child 'apprehended' or received into care. Whilst some workers, who had radical/oppositional discourses and understood the oppression and restriction the risk-preoccupied procedures inflicted upon the young women, felt very troubled by some of the authoritarian actions they had to take and found ways to mitigate against that when they could. In contrast, workers who adhered to a reactionary, neoliberal discourse, that these young women were irresponsible and it was quite correct that they be held to account, had no difficulty in following procedure, reporting concerns or using coercion. These different discourses can be seen in the comments from the current study:

> The issues we try to address to help reduce re-offending are often welfare e.g. accommodation, employment and substance misuse (Radical, oppositional discourse – an underpinning assumption that structural issues contribute to offending)

> (clients need) to be encouraged to empower themselves (Reactionary discourse – clients need to correct their own behaviour)

Similarly, personal moral codes were found by Stanford (2011, p.1520) to be the deciding feature of whether a worker would 'advocate for and protect' service users or 'control and dismiss them'. Empathetic and compassionate practice were features of the 'advocating' group's practice but did not feature in the practice of the 'controlling and dismissing' group. The 'advocating' group also had an understanding of social justice and a belief in the ability of people to change – once again, features missing from the other group. These features depend on a critical understanding of the political and societal context within which people live and make choices, and on a critical understanding of neoliberal explanations of social problems which neglect this context. The newer generation of social workers, so used to neoliberal 'common sense' (Fenton 2014b) may naturally engage in unquestioning compliance with that 'common sense'. Resisting, caring and advocating and building relationships will then feature less and less in social work practice; as Ferguson (2008, p.14) said 'neo- liberal social work … undermines not only radical or structural approaches, but also 'traditional' relationship-based social work'. Morley and Macfarlane (2014, p.352), however, have a hopeful message from their study which found that explicit critical reflection in social work education can lead to the development of moral courage within students, helping them towards 'finding the discretionary space to work towards ethical, socially just outcomes for service users despite practice contexts that might be hostile to critical emancipatory aims'.

The above point seems to be a crucial one – social workers and students need the encouragement to relationship-build in a compassionate and caring way – thus allowing the experience of 'animal pity'. They also need an understanding of social justice (Stanford 2011) and the ability to critically reflect (Morley and Macfarlane 2014), in order to develop moral courage and to want to 'work towards ethical, socially just outcomes for service users' (Morley and Macfarlane 2014). Wiinikka-Lydon (2016) made a convincing case that war veterans should be helped and encouraged to use their experiences of moral injury to critically reflect on the morality of war. Similarly, social workers should be helped to question and critique ideas that underpin a preoccupation with risk assessment and management.

Conclusion

The quantitative element of this study found that the experience of ethical stress, which we equate to moral injury, increased perceptions of an agency being more risk-averse increased. When examining the free text comments made by the respondents one could see that moral injury is experienced by those workers who work in a culture of defensive practice, but want to engage with service users from a different perspective. Workers who focus on relationship building, understanding service users from a lens of social injustice, and practicing within a social welfare context can find working in a highly risk-averse and defensive system antithetical to their moral compass. This is antithetical to the kind of risk-averse, managerial and procedural practice often seen in risk preoccupied agencies and is, of course, completely congruent with social work values and ethics (BASW 2012; IFSW 2012). Therefore, we can define those social workers as having professional and moral integrity. From the results of the current study, in particular the significant relationship between perceived risk aversion and ethical stress, it would appear that most social workers come into this category and are suffering ethical stress and possibly moral injury as a result.

Worryingly, the neoliberal direction of social work practice, and the possibly less critical newer generation of social workers (Fenton 2014b) might contribute to an environment where using ethical stress and moral injury as an impetus towards courageous, innovative practice is increasingly more difficult. It may be that social workers in increasing numbers learn how to assimilate and adapt to a risk-averse, managerial world. To avoid this erosion of professional and moral integrity, social work education should, we would suggest, explicitly highlight and explore concepts of ethical stress leading to moral injury. As such, students can learn to *use* these experiences of moral injury to affect change in practice, rather than learn how to simply cope with them. This in turn should lead to a strengthened social work workforce and a strengthened profession.

References

Barry, M. (2007). *Effective approaches to risk assessment in social work: An international literature review*. Edinburgh: Scottish Government.

Bauman, Z. (1989). *Modernity and the holocaust*. New York, NY: Cornell University Press.

Bauman, Z. (2000). Special essay. Am I my brother's keeper? *European Journal of Social Work, 3*(1), 5–11.

Beresford, P. (2012, April 27). What service users want from social workers. *Community Care*

Blinka, D., & Harris, W. H. (2016). Moral injury in warriors and veterans: The challenge to social work. *Social Work & Christianity, 43*(2), 7–27.

Boudreau, T. (2011). The morally injured. *The Massachusetts Review, 52*(3–4), 746–754.

British Association of Social Workers. (2012). *Code of ethics for social work*. Birmingham, AL: Author.

Broadhurst, K., Hall, C., Wastell, D., White, S., & Pithouse, A. (2010). Risk, instrumentalism and the humane project in social work: Identifying the informal logics of risk management in children's statutory services. *British Journal of Social Work, 40*(4), 1046–1064.

Carson, D., & Bain, A. (2008). *Professional risk and working with people: Decision-making in health, social care and criminal justice*. London: Jessica Kingsley.

Carey, M. (2009). *The social work dissertation*. Maidenhead: McGraw-Hill.

Chenot, D., Benton, A. D., & Kim, H. (2009). Support, peer support, and organizational culture among early career social workers in child welfare services. *Child Welfare, 88*(5), 129–147.

Di Franks, N. N. (2008). Social workers and the NASW Code of Ethics: Belief, behaviour and disjuncture. *Social Work, 53*, 167–176.

Drescher, K. D., Foy, D. W., Kelly, C., Leshner, A., Schutz, K., & Litz, B. (2011). An exploration of the viability and usefulness of the construct of moral injury in war veterans. *Traumatology, 17*(1), 8–13.

Feeley, M., & Simon, J. (1992). The new penology: Notes on the emerging strategy of corrections and its implications. *Criminology, 30*, 449–474.

Fenton, J. (2012). Bringing together messages from the literature on criminal justice social work and 'disjuncture': The importance of helping. *British Journal of Social Work, 42*(5), 941–956.

Fenton, J. (2014a). An analysis of 'ethical stress' in criminal justice social work in Scotland: The place of values. *British Journal of Social Work, 45*(5), 1415–1432.

Fenton, J. (2014b). Can social work education meet the neoliberal challenge head on? *Critical and Radical Social Work, 2*(3), 321–335.

Ferguson, I. (2008). *Reclaiming social work: Challenging neo-liberalism and promoting social justice*. London: Sage.

Finefter-Rosenbluh, I. (2016). Behind the scenes of reflective practice in professional development: A glance into the ethical predicaments of secondary school teachers. *Teaching and Teacher Education, 60*, 1–11.

Fischer, J., & Corcoran, K. (2007). *Measures for clinical practice: A sourcebook* (4th ed.). New York, NY: Oxford University Press.

Frankfurt, S., & Frazier, P. (2016). A review of research on moral injury in combat veterans. *Military Psychology, 28*(5), 318–330.

Gilligan, P. (2007). Well motivated reformists or nascent radicals: How do applicants to the degree in social work see social problems, their origins and solutions? *British Journal of Social Work, 37*(4), 735–760.

Hennessey, R. (2011). *Relationship skills in social work*. London: Sage.

International Federation of Social Workers. (2012) *Statement of ethical principles*. Retrieved from https://ifsw.org/policies/statement-of-ethical-principles/

Johnson, R. B., & Onwuegbuzie, A. J. (2004). Mixed methods research: A research paradigm whose time has come. *Educational Researcher, 33*(7), 14–26.

Jones, C. (2001). Voices from the front line: State social workers and new labour. *British Journal of Social Work, 31*, 547–562.

Jones, O. (2011). *Chavs: Demonization of the working class*. London: Verso.

Joseph Rowntree Foundation. (2014) *Public attitudes towards poverty*. Retrieved from https://www.jrf.org.uk/publications/public-attitudes-towards-poverty

Kemshall, H. (2002). *Risk, social policy and welfare*. Buckingham: OU Press.

Kosny, A., & Eakin, J. (2008). The hazards of helping: Work, mission and risk in non-profit social service organizations. *Health, Risk and Society, 10*, 149–166.

Levinson, M. (2015). Moral injury and the ethics of educational injustice. *Harvard Educational Review, 85*(2), 203–228.

Littlechild, B. (2010). Child protection social work: Risks of fears and fears of risk – Impossible tasks from impossible goals? *Social Policy and Administration., 42*, 662–675.

Litz, B. T., Stein, N., Delaney, E., Lebowitz, L., Nash, W. Pl, Silva, C., & Maguen, Shira (2009). Moral injury and moral repair in war veterans: A preliminary model and intervention strategy. *Clinical Psychology Review, 29*, 696–706.

Munro, E. (2011). *The Munro review of child protection: Final report*. London: TSO.

Murray, C. (1990). *The emerging British underclass*. London: IEA Health and Welfare Unit.

Morley, C., & Macfarlane, S. (2014). Critical social work as ethical social work: Using critical reflection to research students' resistance to neoliberalism. *Critical and Radical Social Work, 2*(3), 337–355.

Pallant, J. (2010). *SPSS survival manual* (4th ed.). Maidenhead: OU Press.

Phillips, D. (2009). Beyond the risk agenda. In S. Green, E. Lancaster, & S. Feasey (Eds.), *Addressing offending behaviour: Context, practice and values* (pp. 172–189). Devon: Willan.

Preston-Shoot, M. (2003). Changing learning and learning change. *Journal of Social Work Practice, 17*(1), 9–23.

Reamer, F. G. (2014). Moral injury in social work. *Social Work Today*. Retrieved from https://www.socialworktoday.com/news/eoe_021814.shtml

Rogowski, S. (2015). From child welfare to child protection/safeguarding: A critical practitioner's view of changing conceptions. *Policies and Practice, Practice, 27*(2), 97–112.

Rudestam, K. E., & Newton, R. R. (2007). *Surviving your dissertation: A comprehensive guide to content and process* (3rd ed.). London: Sage.

Schein, E. H. (2010). *Organisational culture and leadership* (4th ed.). Hoboken: Jossey-Bass.

Scottish Social Services Council (2016). *Code of practice for social services workers and employers*. Dundee: SSSC.

Shay, J. (2014). Moral injury. *Psychoanalytic Psychology, 31*(2), 182–191.

Smith, M. (2011). Reading Bauman for social work. *Ethics and Social Welfare, 5*(1), 2–17.

Stanford, S. N. (2011). Constructing moral responses to risk: A framework for hopeful social work practice. *British Journal of Social Work, 41*, 1514–1531.

Taylor, B. J. (2017). *Decision making, assessment and risk in social work* (3rd ed.). Thousand Oaks, CA: Learning, Kindle Edition.

Taylor, M. (2007). Professional dissonance: A promising concept for clinical social work. *Smith College Studies in Social Work, 77*, 89–99.

Turbett, C. (2014). *Doing radical social work*. Basingstoke: Palgrave Macmillan.

Webb, S. (2006). *Social work in a risk society: Social and political perspectives*. Hampshire: Palgrave MacMillan.

Weinberg, M. (2016). *Pradoxes in social work practice: Mitegating ethical trespass*. Abingdon: Routledge.

Wiinikka-Lydon, J. (2016). Moral injury as inherent political critique: The prophetic possibilities of a new term. *Political Theology, 18*, 219–232.

Woods, N., & Rafaeli, J. S. (2016). *Good cop, bad war*. London: Ebury Press.

Tony Stanley, Surinder Guru and Vicki Coppock

A RISKY TIME FOR MUSLIM FAMILIES: PROFESSIONALISED COUNTER-RADICALISATION NETWORKS

In July 2015, a new statutory duty was sanctioned in the UK for a range of professional practitioners, including social workers, to pay 'due regard to preventing terrorism'. The duty has contributed to a shifting of social work practice and decision-making from the fields of advocacy and promotion of ethics, social justice and human rights, towards risk-work more analogous to that of the security services. Social workers are caught up in pre-emptive risk work, operating in a pre-crime space. Further, an 'ethic of silence' has emerged because social workers are not speaking back or challenging the duty due to the ensnared nature of the dominant securitised discourses, which prevent counter-discourses from emerging. Utilising an autoethnographic approach, this paper shows that the new duty is reorganising and rearranging new networks of practitioners with securitisation a dominant feature, and this significantly affects practice decisions. Latour's actor network theory (ANT) helps us to examine the ethical and practical implications for decision-making. Shifting notions of ethics, rights and as yet unforeseen consequences of PREVENT concern us. This being said, humane and socially just social work practice within the duty is possible; strengths-based risk practices provide practical and ethical ways forward and these are discussed.

Introduction

The *Prevent Duty,* a part of UK's counter-terrorism strategy, was sanctioned in July 2015, and this fundamentally adjusted how a range of UK professional practitioners, including social workers, carry out day-to-day practice, because they now have to pay 'due regard to preventing terrorism' (*Counter Terrorism and Security Act* 2015). This duty has contributed to a shifting of social work practice and decision-making from the fields of advocacy and promotion of social justice and human rights, towards risk-work resembling security services (Petrie 2015). Social workers are working in a pre-crime space in order to prevent terrorist crimes occurring in the first place. In this context, we suggest, the capacity to deliver humane, rights based and socially just statutory social work in England is compromised. Families and extended family members are neglected in the risk-work of extremism and counter-radicalisation practice where an over focus on children and youth dominates at the expense of family, community and societal approaches questioning wider structures of society. The lived experiences of people subject to statutory social work and those working in this emerging area of social work practice are poorly understood and not readily available (Guru 2012b; Stanley & Guru 2015). Moreover, critical debate about this emerging area of work is underdeveloped (Heath-Kelly 2013). This highlights a lack of ethical debate and justice ideals so central to the social work project. With scant practice debate and no empirical studies about practice decision-making, this highlights an important area that needs to be examined.

The paper draws on a set of composite 'at risk' narratives of two families' fathers accused of radicalising their children – concerns about fathers are the main source of referral to children's services. The practice is informed by one of the authors lived ex- perience of doing social work in cases involving actual or potential referrals to Prevent. We show how dominant discourses of 'risk as certainty' are leaving families disadvan- taged, neglected, distrusted and potentially harmed by these new professionalised and securitised networks. Taking an autoethnographic perspective illuminates the way in which families come to be classified, while notions of ethics and debates about human rights rendered unnecessary or redundant.

Below, we provide an overview of *Prevent* and the *Prevent Duty*, in which we describe the law and policy context and explain how 'radicalisation risk' is presented in official discourse. This is followed by a methods discussion where autoethnography and the two composite case narratives are discussed, including our critical reflections. From here we engage further critical debate, opening up the 'black box' of decision-making, and then consider practice implications of the *Prevent Duty*. We expose the way power, discourse and ethics affect and shape decision-making whether to act or not and what this means for families subject to the state's terrorism gaze – something we term 'risk- work' (Horlick-Jones 2005). Finally, we offer some possibilities on ways to work more effectively and ethically in this contentious field.

Prevent overview

In the post-9/11 era, many nation states widened the scope of their counter-terrorism strategies to include policies and practices aimed at the prevention of 'extremism'. *Pre- vent* is the 'preventative strand' of the British government's over-arching *CONTEST* coun- ter-terrorism strategy; its stated aim: to 'stop people becoming terrorists or supporting terrorism' (HM Government 2011, p.6). A key objective of *Prevent* is to 'respond to the ideological challenge of terrorism' by undertaking 'counter-ideological work' designed to ensure that there should be 'no ungoverned spaces in which extremism is allowed to flourish' (HM Government 2011, p.9). The government has defined 'extremism' as 'vocal or active opposition to fundamental British values including, democracy, the rule of law, individual liberty and mutual respect and tolerance of different faiths and beliefs' (HM Government 2011, p.107). 'Radicalisation' is understood as the process whereby people either become terrorists or come to support terrorism. In this process 'extremist ideas' are propagated and disseminated by 'extremist activists' who 'radicalise' persons who are 'vulnerable' to such messages. Therefore, identifying the nature of 'vulnerability' is seen as a crucial means of preventing 'radicalisation' (HM Government 2011).

The government perceives the strongest threat to security to come from 'Al Qa'ida and like-minded groups' and so defines the ideology of 'Islamist extremism' as referring not to 'traditional religious' practices, but to 'a distorted interpretation of Islam', which betrays Islam's peaceful principles…' This ideology is considered the most dangerous because its adherents' deem Western intervention in Muslim-majority countries as a 'war on Islam', creating a narrative of 'them' and 'us' (Cabinet Office 2013, p.1). Certain groups of people are positioned as particularly vulnerable to radicalisation, primarily children, who are considered at risk of being 'groomed' to adopt such radical ideology (Stanley & Guru 2015). Thus, following the introduction of the *Counter Terrorism and Security Act 2015 (CTSA 2015)* the social work role in protecting children was extended to include 'children who are or might be radicalising'. The *CTSA 2015* introduced a statutory duty for all public sector workers to have 'due regard to the need to prevent people from being drawn into terrorism' (Section 26). The *Prevent Duty* became effective from 1 July 2015. It is underpinned by Statutory Guidance (Section 29), which states that all education, health and social care staff must:

- have a good understanding of *Prevent*
- be trained to recognise a child or young person's vulnerability to being drawn into terrorism
- be aware of programmes that can deal with this issue
- make appropriate referrals to *Channel*

Local Safeguarding Children Boards are now required to ensure that practitioners work to protect children from 'radicalisation risk'. They remind practitioners to be alert to any reason for concern in the child's life at home or elsewhere; this includes awareness of the expression of extremist views. Fundamental 'British values' are promoted as a mechanism to help keep children safe and promote their welfare. Thus, social workers are expected to work in pre-emptory ways to help prevent radicalisation. The vulnerability assessment framework is the main tool for counter terrorism police to determine levels of risk. Focusing on individual traits and vulnerability factors, an individual approach is encouraged (Coppock & McGovern 2014). The vulnerability-based approach that counter-terror measures have adopted is encroaching on the thought processes of young people because it focuses on individuals at risk or potentially posing a risk to others. Radicalisation risk categories and cases emerge.

All government (and related) employees are now under the umbrella of the new *Prevent Duty*, thus accountability and legitimacy of certain activities, like information sharing, is generally unquestioned. As *Prevent* has been rolled out throughout the public sector, very few voices of practitioner resistance are evident. Teachers have demonstrated some resistance, concerned about both the welfare of their pupils as well as their own expertise and capacity to identify extremism, but elsewhere there is a general silence, partly borne of confusion and apathy (The Guardian 2016). In the social work arena, a profession given to anti-oppressive practice, awareness is only tentatively emerging, and there is scant practice guidance about how to address the *Prevent Duty* (Stanley & Guru 2015). Given the confidentiality and the guarded nature of cases surrounding Prevent and Channel, the day-to-day social work practice is off limits to researchers and any wider debate. And rather like the workings of an aircraft black-box, the work is carried out in private spaces and then rendered semi-public through a range of file recordings and court documents. Thus, understanding the various discursive influences that are at play in practice has been off limits. We therefore, draw upon autoethnography as a way of exploring and reflecting upon social work practice decisions as this has research relevance.

Methodology

Actor network theory (ANT) offers a method to help open the private 'black-boxes' of practice, by explaining the relationships between people, things and the various forms of codified knowledge that circulate between and around them (Latour 2005). ANT argues that order is provisionally secured through the various associations between human and nonhuman actants. Further, interactions are regarded as being at the crossroads of trajectories already in flow, existing practices and approaches of work are already set in motion. To secure a *new* provisional order the various actors have to accept their position within the network. This is achieved through a process of enrolment. Enrolment is the result of the interactions whereby someone becomes interested in something. Thus, interests drive the sorts of knowledge claims able to be made and accepted, while iteratively shaping those very interests. According to Callon and Law (1982) actors' interests are the outcome of negotiations and interactions: thus, they become enrolled to accept the new provisional order *is in* their best interest. Following this idea, actors' interests are an outcome, a socially produced experience that is actually generated from social negotiations and interactions. Police reports and evidence documents, as part of this network, play a crucial role in practice. They are mostly regarded as true and accepted as fact and serve to cohere order since actors come to perceive their interests in preserving order (van de Luitgaarden 2011).

Autoethnography offers a qualitative approach that honours subjectivity and suggests a particular way of practitioners and researchers 'being in the research' (McGibbon, Peter, & Gallop 2010). It builds on and extends ethnographic and autobiographic research methods by inviting the researchers' subjective experience to be placed at the centre of the inquiry. It encourages the researcher or practitioner to be extraordinarily reflective and self-aware about the discursive messaging and structural influences that impact and thus inform a range of critical questions about the role of certain ideas and ideologies operating alongside dominant narratives (Gupta 2017). Autoethnographic accounts use a first person narrative of experience, and the researcher engages with the text in order that the researcher's interpretations of the narratives can reveal new ideas about the course of study. Phenomena and experience often off limits to external researchers becomes accessible and the reflective capacity of the practitioner is a vehicle through which debate and questioning can rest and emerge. Denshire (2013) argues this helps us to speak back, and possibly speak differently, about professional life and helps us understand how professional practice is actually made up, occupied, and enacted. Gupta (2017) termed this 'learning from others' – and this is of research relevance.

The ethics of research need some explanation. Gaining traditional ethics committee approval is highly problematic in this area of practice (Guru2012b). Is it ethical to go back to previous work places and closed cases to seek consent? Whose consent speaks on behalf of a composition of mixed narratives? And by doing this are we identifying the local authorities where these people reside? (Gupta 2017). Drawing on composite narratives is used to respect confidentiality while offering insights into the lived experience for these difficult to reach populations (Gupta 2017). Names, ages and family composition have been changed, as have locations. Contributing to practice informed knowledge from a practitioner wisdom perspective is a contribution to social justice and therefore a worthwhile activity for social workers (Guru 2012b).

Narratives are never neutral but interpretational, and the author tells the story as they see it. Ethical telling is an important aspect of this work and we have maintained confidentiality by anonymising details about participants and used fictitious names, so a protection, as far as we can, is afforded to our participants. We have respectfully depicted out subjects, and stayed aware of the potential misuse of interpretative power. Care was taken to offer the narratives in an accessible, respectful and useful way. Field notes made by Stanley, as a practitioner, provided the main source for the narratives. Having an academic interest in 'matters of risk' these cases were a rich ground of social risk issues. He recalls that writing about this unfolding area of work would be difficult and ethically fraught. It is not common for practitioners to write directly about practice, and senior managers are often cautious about such activity. As the work was unfolding, Stanley was advised to not publicise the practice challenges he was facing. Autoethnography helps to overcome this problem because it provides a way to reflexively debate practice from the perspective of the social worker.

The narrative of parents in no way signals a lack of attention to the experience of children growing up in homes where violence and abuse occur. We are aware of cases where a small number of children have been subjected to months of ritualistic abuse through forced watching of degrading and violent beheading videos, and quite rightly issues of mental health were assessed and alternative arrangements for children made. But these cases are rare, and should not be considered the norm. However, parents convicted of terrorist-related activities released from prison or being associated with a banned or proscribed extremist group triggers enough concern for the state to act. Important questions follow. How is risk being assessed in and with these families? What gets drawn on in the making of a risk analysis that these children require statutory social work intervention? What is the social work task here? How has 'the duty' affected the practice of statutory social workers and managers? Is the practice undertaken consistent with professional ideals of upholding rights and being socially just? Two autoethnographic composite cases are offered next. These offer a window through which a consideration of social work decision-making in cases can be critically considered and engaged with.

Mr Malik and family

At a Multi-Agency Public Protection Arrangement (MAPPA) meeting, Mr Malik's case was discussed. He was a 40-year old man, due for release from prison with licence conditions due to end later that year. He was convicted for the distribution of banned material, promoting terrorism, and fundraising to support a banned radical group. Mr Mailk has 4 children, all under the age of 10. They are all home schooled. There was no history of social services involvement. His wife led the children's education. Police, without clear evidence, reported concerns that the children were being exposed to radicalising jihadist ideologies. Some information suggested that the wider family were 'likely to be involved'.

The social worker met with the family alongside the allocated probation officer and police officer. A number of joint home visits followed. Mr Malik allowed the social worker to meet with the children on two occasions, but would not allow them to talk to anyone else, like the family doctor or housing officer. The case was classified under s17 of the Children Act 1989, and the work undertaken within a voluntary consensual manner. A month went by, and Mr Malik told the social worker he did not want to continue the working arrangements. Mr and Mrs Malik declined the offer of any further support and said that they were concerned that the work lacked a clear purpose and they said that they did not see their children to be in harm's way or having needs that could not be met by the family. The case was closed. It was difficult to draw any conclusions based on the brief period of work. Senior managers from probation and police asked for a review of the case, insisting that the children were 'at risk'.

Our reflections

The Malik family found themselves in a maelstrom of growing anxiety around terrorism risk and the limits of statutory power by probation and police services. Mr Malik kept within the law, and by not attending proscribed rallies or banned meetings, limited the state's eye over the family. However, the police's enrolment of children's services initiated a new set of work for the family. Social workers and police collaborated prior to setting up meetings with the family. Early presentations about the children being 'at risk' were potent and influential because the onus then fell to social workers to prove or establish that the children were not. Enrolment by social workers into the police construction of events preceded meeting the family. The family declined a working relationship and did not agree that the children were at risk. The police reports were influential as they provided a documented form of evidence that the state had 'legitimacy' to act on and which the social workers could not question. Ideas of human rights and justice for the family were silenced in debates about protecting the children from what was described as 'ideological forms of abuse'. The parents acted assertively and proved quite knowledgeable and legally aware of their rights to bring the intervention to an end in this event.

Mr Shabir and family

Mr Shabir is 50-year old father of six children and he was released from prison three years ago. He was convicted of promoting terrorist offences and fundraising to support a proscribed group. Mr Shabir was convicted because he was believed to be associating with a terrorist organisation in Syria, and for attending rallies led by a proscribed group. His oldest son is currently in prison for similar offences. He has six children aged three to nineteen. The five younger are all home schooled. Mr Shabir refused to allow social workers to meet his children; however, he did agree to meet the social workers on a number of occasions. He explained that he knew the legal situation and it was 'his right' to bring his children up in the ways of Sharia law and that 'education was a right and a goal for his children'. After a referral was made to social services, the social worker approached a community group who advocated for families in similar situations, and was told by senior police colleagues that community or advocacy groups needed to be on 'an approved list', and so this particular agency could not be used. It was quite difficult for the social worker to offer any tangible support or help to the family. It was also difficult to determine that the children were in harm's way simply because they had attended rallies with their father. Mr Shabir's lawyer wrote to Children's Services advising that the family had withdrawn consent to work together pursuant to s17. Legal advice was to seek an assessment order for the initial assessment of risks of radicalisation by multi-agency safeguarding bodies, and to elevate the matter to a child protection (s47) enquiry where there is a significant harm, as this would dispense with parental consent. The social worker argued that there was not enough evidence of harm. The case was closed. The family left the jurisdiction and were last reported to be in Turkey, probably on route to the Middle East.

Our reflections

Balancing a family's right to private life is pitted against safeguarding duties and delivering the *Prevent Duty*, making the social work role difficult. Social workers are pressured to make the 'right decisions', and this may not always feel just or right for the family; in this case pressure from legal colleagues and managers to err on the side of caution was balanced by the social worker, who argued for proportionality. These actors attempted to enrol the social worker. But what are the implications for less confident workers, or new graduates? Is enrolment into a new provisional order more likely? How does the family's political involvement and political interest in the war in the Middle East affect decision-making? In this case it was considered by the social worker, but argued against by the manager as another sign of risk for the children. The police fed information directly to the social worker and manager, again heightening the risk argument. Young people became simultaneously 'risky' and 'at risk' and this further encouraged a child rescue approach, giving legitimacy for statutory action. In both the above cases, the family became a target for intervention because the father had convictions for terrorist offences. The family is constructed and presented as untrustworthy by managers and legal advisers rather than as a resource to be worked with. The heads of household here had committed (new) terrorism offences and served (or serving) their sentences – and although they were subsequently law abiding, they were nevertheless deemed (potentially) risky of transmitting political values on to their children. It was here, in the fold of socialisation that social workers were required to intervene and decide to limit and engage with the families' political agency, with the aim of instilling a different set of values based on 'Western democracies'. The practice of early intervention into the political realm and agency of families and children, however, poses serious questions about the nature and quality of such democratic principles in the name of liberty and equality while simultaneously going against the grain of anti-oppressive practice.

Discussion – it's a risky time for Muslim families

The bid to identify 'suspected victims' of 'radicalisation' means probing into feelings and beliefs of people and suspecting the family: this is an impossible position from where social workers base their risk decisions. Unlike the majority of other child abuse casework, in these cases there is often a lack of material evidence such as videos or signifiers of group belonging. Social workers are asked to form a view on the possibility that the process of radicalisation maybe or is, indeed, actually happening. The counter-terrorism measures introduced since 2001, including the *Prevent* and *Channel* programmes, mean that there is a monitoring of certain families, their activities, home lives, school lives as well as the work undertaken by health and social work institutions – all now subject to new forms of professionalised responses and sets of surveillance, all channelling families to adopt British values and British ways of life. In this context, Muslim families experience a heightened state of securitisation. They do not have to be found to be committing any crimes; that they are Muslims is sufficient reason for them to be represented as 'dangerous' and 'risky'. A 'panoptical gaze' produces new networks of professionals who form to tackle radicalisation risk. Thus, professionalised responses to risk are legitimised – while families are more likely to be seen as 'pariahs than partners' (Tobis 2013). The Malik children were classified as children in need (pursuant to s17, Children Act 1989), and pressure grew from other actors in the network to reclassify them to child protection (s47) because the family withdrew their cooperation. A legitimising argument is offered, and many workers would have been enrolled in this change of status. Stanley held what he describes as 'an ethical line'. He argued it was family's right to withdraw (under s17), and only new evidence or new concerns should initiate a reclassification.

Referrals to children's services aimed at planning for high risk situations are producing risk identities for the state to monitor; newly formed professionalised networks emerge. Such measures have been criticised for their pathologising and alienating effects, for the increased surveillance and intrusion of privacy and for the erosion of democratic rights and liberties for Muslim people (Breen-Smyth 2014; Choudhury & Fenwick 2011; Coppock & McGovern 2014; Hickman, Thomas, Silvestri, & Nickels 2011; Kundnani 2012; McGovern 2010; Ragazzi 2016). Moreover, these practices of restriction and surveillance form a way of reinforcing Western hegemony – in Gramsci's terms, a 'predominance' gained through consent, 'popularisation', and diffusion, rather than through force. They have historical resonance with colonial practices.

This form of subjection resulted from the need of the coloniser to control resistance and insurrection of the colonised, for example the 'Indian Mutiny' (India 1857), the Sioux Uprising (America 1862) or Jandamarra's War (Australia 1873) which threatened and fought against colonial rulers. In face of the fear and anxiety of rebellion, it was necessary to cast them off as 'abject people' (Tyler 2013), represented with disgust, contempt and revulsion, which the negative imagery and the coercive ideology about the colonised as the 'barbarian', 'savage', so redolent of Orientalism, did quite successfully. The colonised had to be ruled through every part of their social and cultural life: this meant a full repression, reform and reconstitution of their physical, cultural and political identities that dehumanised and illegalised their existence, made them moral outcasts.

The insistence upon instilling 'British values' and entrenching 'Western democracy' through programmes such as *Prevent* and *Channel* represent neo-colonial techniques of suppression and repression. The discourse about '*the Muslim community*' and its 'Islamic inspired terrorism', despite the murmurings about its heterogeneity, is largely configured by the state as a homogenous group. Whilst categorisations of the 'good' and 'bad' Muslim (Bettiza2015) have been variously constructed, it is the image of the 'Islamic terrorist' and its perceived sympathisers that predominate as 'the community'. As Jacoby (2004) points out, such discourses about the failure of the 'other' to inculcate 'Britishness' are anxious about the attack on 'our values' and 'our way of life', but say nothing about politics or foreign policy decisions and related issues. In focusing on cultures and psychologies, it denies the *politics* of radicalisation that is fundamental to an understanding of the rebellion that is terrorism (Haslam 2016). This resonates in the Malik case when senior managers and lawyers argued for a redefining of the case to be 'higher risk' despite any new evidence to support this.

Constructed as distrustful, the Shabir and Malik families were closed off from practice decision-making, constructed as not able to protect – thus *posing* a risk. The professional and securitised network takes a legitimised leadership role in the work with a dualism of perpetrator and victim operating. Thus, child rescue discourse enters and is unproblematic. A new discourse operates. He is no longer a child, thus no longer constructed as 'at risk,' – rather he is now an adult and so an active perpetrator. Data sharing is unquestioned, with notions of ethics and rights easily ignored or disregarded. Mostly this means police seeking or providing information *to* social workers. However, information from police and counter security officers is always partial – they do not release everything. This practice reinforces and reimagines the social work task into networks of security to search out and manage those deemed deviant, sorely challenging the historical alliance of social work with social activism, justice and radical traditions. Further, the issues concerned with privacy and confidentiality are set aside without debate, as the unassailable evocation of counter terrorism and child rescue discourses drawn on to offer powerful legitimation of state processes, with scant debate about negative effects or consequences (Stanley & Guru 2015).

The *Prevent Duty* has produced serious implications for delivering the ethical and humane promise of social work. In the current climate of heightened anxieties around preventing the radicalisation of Muslim children and youth, and the concomitant denigration and demonisation of Muslim communities and Islam, social work practice is problematic. The use of the word 'radical' is now ubiquitous as a negative term synonymous with fear of terrorist violence, and is almost exclusively associated with Muslims and Islam. Yet, we should be mindful that the core principles and values that underpin the social work profession internationally have their origins in the *radical* social work tradition of the 1970s (Bailey & Brake 1975). Indeed, the *radical* social work ideals of empowerment, rights and social justice are formally institutionalised in all of the official statements, definitions and Codes of Practice of leading social work organisations and in curricula for social work education and training worldwide.

Social work is a practice-based profession and an academic discipline that promotes social change and development, social cohesion and the empowerment and liberation of people. Principles of social justice, human rights, collective responsibility and respect for diversities are central to social work. Underpinned by theories of social work, social science, humanities and indigenous knowledge, social work engages people and structures to address life challenges and address wellbeing. (International Federation of Social Workers [IFSW] 2014)

In effect, this means that if social workers are not identifying and challenging discrimination towards the Muslim children, young people and families with whom they work then they are not practising social work according to the principles and values laid down by the IFSW. Holding an ethical line is not easy. Stanley found it uncomfortable to be in opposition to colleagues who argued for removal of children from the Malik and Shabir homes. Augments to remove children from these homes are easy to make. But such is not practice socially just or in line with the international federation's definition of social work.

Radical social work theory illuminated a long-disguised reality; that social work is, and always has been, an inherently political activity. This means that unless the world-wide political context surrounding social work is both recognised and the issues made visible, social workers will not understand the significance of changes to law, policy and practice and their impact on the children, families and communities with whom they work. Moreover, they risk exacerbating and further perpetuating inequality and oppressive practices (Thompson & Thompson2008). Clearly, through its counter-terrorism strategy, the British state is currently driving law, policy and practice in ways that are inconsistent with the professional norms and core values of the social work profession. Such moral and professional dilemmas are by no means new as there has always been a longstanding and intrinsic tension for social work in regulating the state/child/family nexus (Parton 2014a, 2014b). However, these tensions have intensified considerably in recent times. The introduction of the duty, the impact of securitisation and the relocation and reassembling of practice into the pre-crime space is rapidly transforming what it means to do social work in the neoliberal era (Stanley & Guru 2015). We are arguing for new forms of practice to counter the securitisation dominance that featured in the Shabir and Malik cases.

Strengths-based methods – more humane ways forward

For many families, the offer of *Prevent* has been taken up and found helpful. Others have declined this offer, and a referral to children social care follows. Too often, in the name of helping, we remove a child from what we define as an unsafe household. Risk aversion is influential – and we are driven and encouraged to avoid risk taking measures – *just in case*! Families are not helped when such practices dominate. They tend to be enrolled into accepting the professionalised and securitised version of order. This being said, there are humane strengths-based approaches that we can draw on to counter this dominance. For example, the Signs of Safety approach (Turnell & Edwards 1999) takes a comprehensive approach to analysing danger, existing strengths and safety/protective factors and future safety and utilises a simple judgement scaling process to involve all participants (Stanley & Mills 2014; Turnell & Edwards 1999). This practice supports risk as an assemblage of views that is socially constructed and positioned – altered and adjusted by the range of actions social workers and families take. Risk is understood as something fluid and shifting, and something that can be managed and lived with. A simple but effective 0–10 scaling question (where 0 means dangerous and 10 means safe enough) is used to invite risk interpretations from everyone involved. Family members and practitioners provide a score. This practice, simple but effective, invites family views to be considered alongside practitioners. Power is shared and scores more concerning are talked through with those that see risk as less worrying. Solutions and decisions to help manage risk are co-produced. Different views are thus not problematic, rather invitational to review what and how views are formed. Signs of safety can be used with individuals, groups or whole communities and this methodology offers a powerful tool for social workers to use in this area of radicalisation or violent extremism. Stanley's experience with the Malik family shows that this method offers a way to balance danger and hope. It offers a visual tool for the Malik family to help them to understand what worries the social worker. Stanley found this helped engage the families. This helped him to continue to assess the attitudes, beliefs, subtleties and nuances of the family system.

The 'signs of safety' practice methodology offers a coherent language about risk assessment and family strengths and is a practice framework that can traverse disciplines. Police, social work and health can employ the same assessing framework and work collaboratively with a shared understanding of what is most worrying, most risky, and engage the resources on hand in family and community to help offset this. Cases can be analysed using a consistent practice methodology that multiple agencies share, and following a case mapping, the risk statements become a very useful vehicle for the planning of next steps. Definitions of risk can be conceptually and practically mapped at the interface of police and social work practice, with children and their families, to strengthen the case analysis and to inform the social work plans about what needs to happen next. The 'signs of safety' approach offers a coherent and logical methodology for risk analysis practice within and across the disciplines of social work and police.

The Family Group Conference (FGC) is another practice method for working humanely with radicalisation concerns (Stanley and Gunstone 2016). FGC offers a restorative intervention approach for working with risk. This is a family-focused restorative model where the resources within and around the family are drawn on to harness safety and strengths to help children *and* families. It provides a facilitated space for families to locate solutions and options to help keep their young people and children safer. This offers a way to reintroduce trust as the private family time is not part of the states working sphere; and a new black box is part of the work but one that helps to facilitate debate and decisions led by the family and then presented to the social workers/managers. This offers meaningful and respectful power sharing and through finding and building solutions together, professionalised security networks are balanced by family networks producing plans that help to drive safer options for their children. The family's reality is a balanced and powerful antidote to the discursive dominance and silencing effects produced by securitising networks.

The Malik and Shabir families were not offered this. The testing out by other family members is a worthwhile and ethical activity for social work. Trying to determine how belief systems and ideological views may turn into more sinister activities is practically impossible for social workers. However, family members challenging each other on ideas and beliefs that they see problematic for their own is a core part of the FGC process. This method is now being used in parts of the country to do just that (Stanley & Gunstone 2016).

Conclusion

The present climate is less than conducive to the form and quality of social work practice that the IFSW advocates for. In such an unsympathetic environment, it is beholden on social workers to reflect critically on their contradictory position as both allies of oppressed Muslim families and communities and potential 'agents of the state'. As Guru (2012a, p.1155) argues, 'social workers and social work educators have a duty to raise awareness of the environment in which families affected by counter-terrorism live and become familiar with their social, psychological/emotional, political, economic and religious context [in order that] social workers can be better equipped to negotiate trusting relationships built upon respect, warmth, compassion and non-judgemental attitudes'. Hence social workers need to show awareness of dilemmas presented by wider political problems of foreign policy, poverty and deprivation (Bywaters, Brady, Sparks, & Bos 2014). It has never been more imperative that social work resists the neo-liberal straight jacket, fights back and reconnects with its intellectual, ethical and justice roots. In so doing, it will be more likely that the principles of equality and social justice that symbolise what it means to 'do social work' can be reclaimed and social workers freed to deliver humane, respectful, rights-based practice decisions for Muslim children, families and communities.

References

Bailey, R., & Brake, M. (Eds.). (1975). *Radical social work*. London: Edward Arnold.

Bettiza, G. (2015). Constructing civilisations: Embedding and reproducing the 'Muslim world' in American foreign policy practices and institutions since 9/11. *Review of International Studies, 41*, 575–600.

Breen-Smyth, M. (2014). Theorising the "suspect community": Counterterrorism, security practices and the public imagination. *Critical Studies on Terrorism, 7*(2), 223–240.

Bywaters, P., Brady, G., Sparks, T., & Bos, E. (2014). Child welfare inequalities: New evidence, further questions. *Child & Family Social Work. 21*(3), 369–380. doi:10.1111/cfs.12154

Cabinet Office. (2013). *Tackling extremism in the UK: Report from the Prime Minster's task force on tackling radicalisation and extremism, HM government*. Retrieved March 1, 2017, from https://www.gov.uk/government/uploads/system/uploads/attachment_data/file/263181/ETF_FINAL.pdf

Callon, M., & Law, J. (1982). On Interests and their Transformation: Enrolment and Counter-Enrolment. *Social Studies of Science, 12*(4), 615–625.

Choudhury, T., & Fenwick, H. (2011). *The impact of counter-terrorism measures on Muslim communities*. London: Equality and Human Rights Commission.

Coppock, V., & McGovern, M. (2014). 'Dangerous minds'? Deconstructing counter-terrorism discourse, radicalisation and the 'psychological vulnerability' of Muslim children and young people in Britain. *Children & Society, 28*, 242–256.

Denshire, S. (2013). *Autoethnography*. Retrieved March 1, 2017, from http://www.sagepub.net/isa/resources/pdf/Autoethnography.pdf

The Guardian. (2016, March 28). *Teachers back motion calling for Prevent strategy to be scrapped*. Retrieved February 9, 2017, from https://www.theguardian.com/politics/2016/mar/28/teachers-nut-back-motion-calling-prevent-strategy-radicalisation-scrapped

Gupta, A. (2017). Learning from others: An autoethnographic exploration of children and families social work, poverty and the capability approach. *Qualitative Social Work, 16*(4), 449–464. doi:10.1177/1473325015620946

Guru, S. (2012a). Under siege: Families of counter-terrorism. *British Journal of Social Work, 42*(6), 1151–1173.

Guru, S. (2012b). Reflections on research: Families affected by counterterrorism in the UK. *International Social Work, 55*(5), 689–703.

Haslam, N. (2016). Concept creep: Psychology's expanding concepts of harm and pathology. *Psychological Inquiry, 27*(1), 1–17. doi:10.1080/1047840X.2016.1082418

Heath-Kelly, C. (2013). Counter-terrorism and the counterfactual: Producing the 'radicalisation' discourse and the UK PREVENT strategy. *The British Journal of Politics and International Relations, 15*(3), 394–415.

Hickman, M., Thomas, L., Silvestri, S., & Nickels, N. (2011). *'Suspect communities'? Counterterrorism policy, the press, and the impact on Irish and Muslim communities in Britain, ESRC, London Metropolitan University*. Retrieved September 1, 2015, from http://openaccess.city.ac.uk/8735/

HM Government. (2011). *Prevent Strategy*. London: HM Government. Retrieved March 1, 2017, from https://www.gov.uk/government/uploads/system/uploads/attachment_data/file/97976/prevent-strategy-review.pdf

HM Government. (2015). *Counter Terrorism and Security Act, 2015*. London: The Stationery Office.

Horlick-Jones, T. (2005). On risk work: Professional discourse and everyday action. *Health Risk and Society, 7*(3), 293–307.

International Federation of Social Workers. (2014). *Global definition of social work*. Retrieved February 9, 2017, from http://ifsw.org/policies/definition-of-social-work/

Jacoby, T. (2004). The 'Muslim menace'. *Violence and the DePolitcising Elements of the New Culturalism, Journal of Muslim Minority Affairs, 30*(2), 167–181.

Kundnani, A. (2012). Radicalisation: The journey of a concept. *Race and Class, 54*(2), 3–25.

Latour, B. (2005). *Reassembling the social: An introduction to social life*. Oxford: Oxford University Press.

McGibbon, E., Peter, E., & Gallop, R. (2010). An Institutional ethnography of nurses' stress. *Qualitative Health Research, 20*(10), 1353–1378. doi:10.1177/1049732310375435

McGovern, M. (2010) *'Countering terror or counter-productive? Comparing irish and british muslim experiences of counter- insurgency law and policy'*. Report of a symposium held in Cultúrlann McAdam Ó Fiaich, Falls Road, Belfast, 23–24 June 2009. Retrieved January 6, 2012, from www.edgehill.ac.uk/documents/news/CounteringTerror.pdf

Parton, N. (2014a). Social work, child protection and politics: Some critical and constructive reflections. *British Journal of Social Work., 44*(7), 2042–2056. doi:10.1093/bjsw/bcu091

Parton, N. (2014b). *The politics of child protection. Contemporary developments and future directions*. Basingstoke: Palgrave Macmillan.

Petrie, S. (2015). How UK anti-terror guidance could violate children's human rights. *The Conversation*. Retrieved December 22, 2017, from https://theconversation.com/how-uk-anti-terror-guidance-could-violate-childrens-human-rights-45013

Ragazzi, F. (2016). Suspect community or suspect category? The impact of counter-terrorism as 'policed multiculturalism'. *Journal of Ethnic and Migration Studies, 42*(5), 724–741. doi:10.1080/1369183X.2015.1121807

Stanley, T., & Gunstone, L. (2016). *Family networks can be a critical resource in social work response to 'violent extremism'*. Retrieved May 19, 2017, from http://www.communitycare.

co.uk/2016/04/27/family-networks-can-critical-resource-social-work-response-violent-extremism/

Stanley, T., & Guru, S. (2015). Childhood radicalisation risk: An emerging practice issue. *Practice, 27*(5), 353–366. doi:10.1080/09503153.2015.1053858

Stanley, T., & Mills, R. (2014). 'Signs of safety'practice at the health and children's social care interface. *Practice, 26*(1), 23–36. doi:10.1080/09503153.2013.867942

Thompson, S., & Thompson, N. (2008). *The Critically Reflective Practitioner*. Basingstoke: Palgrave Macmillan.

Tobis, D. (2013). *From pariahs to partners: How parents and their allies changed New York City's child welfare system*. London: Oxford University Press.

Turnell, A., & Edwards, S. (1999). *Signs of safety: A solution and safety oriented approach to child protection casework*. New York, NY: Norton.

Tyler, I. (2013). *Revolting subjects: Social abjection and resistance in neoliberal Britain*. London: Zed Books.

van de Luitgaarden, G. (2011). *Contextualising judgements and decisions in child protection practice at the point of first referral Journal of Social Intervention, 20*, 24–40.

Alessandro Sicora ⓘ

REFLECTIVE PRACTICE, RISK AND MISTAKES IN SOCIAL WORK

Reflection on mistakes is a powerful source for more effective decision-making and action. Mistakes are inevitable and security has also costs and not only benefits. So, in the frame of appropriate error prevention systems, social workers should pay special attention to latent errors and risks, find immediate measures to repair and limit harm and learn to prevent similar events in the future. Nonetheless, exploration and experimentation are needed when previous attempts made using ordinary strategies failed. In doing so, social workers can greatly benefit from their colleagues' feedbacks. Blame culture is probably the main obstacle to expressing and listening to affirmative and useful feedback on mistakes. 'Smart questions', reflective frameworks, reflective friends, concise reflective writing are some of the easiest and more effective strategies aimed at improving the quality of decision-making on the basis of new learning developed by reflecting on mistakes.

Introduction: we do not learn from our mistakes, we learn from reflecting on them

Making mistakes is an inevitable part of social work, as is any other human activity. Social workers plan a series of actions in order to achieve certain goals for the benefit of their service users, but sometimes the outcomes are far from the intended ones and, in some cases, they make situations worse, not better.

Professional mistakes, especially in sensitive areas like child protection, may produce many troubles to individuals and families, as well as the practitioners who made them. Moreover, superficial analysis of what happened may even weaken the core legitimation of the profession and raise intense public condemnation of the 'guilty'.

Blame culture, leading to individual workers being publicly punished in unhelpful ways is probably the strongest obstacle to the spreading of a different and more beneficial perspective. To repair and prevent mistakes, social workers should instead recognise that something 'went wrong', reflect and understand what happened. At the same time, they should also take responsibility for their own actions when the latter, always together with the acts of other people, lead to something negative. Creating a culture of responsibility benefits service users, practitioners and organisations. It implicates the will to see, not to keep one's eyes closed, and this may lead to detect latent risks and prevent graver failures and harm. Some mistakes, in fact, are like alarm signals making visible systemic fragility and the risk of disastrous events in the future. Would it be wise to allow an airplane to take off when its flight instruments show there is something wrong? Social work organisations are very complex systems where any single sentinel event is of vital importance to enhance the service quality.

There is another problem that makes the discourse on professional mistakes in social work even more difficult and intricate: health and social care professions apply scientific knowledge and practice wisdom and use strategies and techniques that can never guarantee an absolute certainty of success because of the complexity and uniqueness of every human being and the continuous change of the environmental and social conditions. These professions are involved in a never-ending process of trial-and-error applied to those unique situations where no known remedy works. In these cases, exploration is the only way to really help service users when previous attempts made using ordinary and normal strategies have failed. But where are the limits of this exploration, and how is possible to solve the inevitable ethical dilemmas arising from the daily practice? Exploration and experimentation may have a cost; failure has a cost, too, so what to do?

In fact, when talking about costs and benefits of decision-making in social work, it is important to highlight that errors may have a cost (that is, it may harm someone) but error and risk prevention systems, too, are costly. For example, how to have absolutely no risk of child abuse and maltreatment in any family? The extreme solution would be to remove all children from their families. Of course, this extreme solution is absolutely unethical and would even lead to further and worse risks. In other words, it could be efficient, but at an enormous and unacceptable cost. So, how to balance the cost of making mistakes with the cost of being totally risk averse?

The purpose of this article is to investigate the complex field of risk and mistakes in social work and highlight reflective practice as the most promising area in which to find some of the answers to the above questions. Firstly, error and professional mistakes will be defined, in addition to error prevention systems and their functions being described. Secondly, risk and latent error will be considered in the light of the so-called 'Swiss Cheese' model designed by Reason (1990). Explaining the dynamics of errors and failures, this model demonstrates that any negative outcome is always the final result of a chain of events and actions whose responsibility is never related to a single subject. Scapegoating is a very human but also ineffective solution. Blaming and punishing represent a false way out and do not solve the real problem. Finally, it will be argued that reflection on errors, as a form of reflective practice, is a powerful means of improving the quality of social work and create innovation where 'normal' and 'common' solutions are ineffective.

Making mistakes in social work

Everyday social workers meet their service users, examine their stories and living conditions, assess them and carefully plan appropriate actions in order to engage, 'people and structures to address life challenges and enhance wellbeing' (International Association of Social Workers [IFSW] & International Association of School of Social Work [IASSW] 2014). Despite this, after the plan is implemented, the intended outcome is sometimes not achieved. In other words, there could be something erroneous in the assessment or in the intervention (or in both).

In his seminal work 'The human error' (1990), Reason defines *error, mistake and other connected concepts*:

> Error will be taken as a generic term to encompass all those occasions in which a planned sequence of mental or physical activities fails to achieve its intended outcome, and when these failures cannot be attributed to the intervention of some chance agency. (...) Mistakes may be defined as deficiencies or failures in the judgemental and/or inferential processes involved in the selection of an objective or in the specification of the means to achieve it, irrespective of whether or not the actions directed by this decision-scheme run according to plan (Reason 1990, p.9).

Even if in everyday language, as well as in this article, error and mistake are often used as synonymous, Reason (1990, p.13) considers the second as a form of the first, occurring during the cognitive stage of planning. Lapses and slips are located in the stages of storage and execution, respectively.

From a different perspective, Schulz (2010, p.17) gives a different and interesting definition focused on the *experience of error*, which is the 'experience of rejecting as false a belief *we ourselves* [original emphasis] once thought was true – regardless of that belief's actual relationship to reality, or whether such a relationship can ever be determined'. When social workers have this experience they vividly encounter the conflicting perspectives often emerging in the field they are engaged day after day. What an individual or a collective considers right now could have been considered wrong in the past and vice versa. This happens because understanding of good practice evolves, but also because, for very good reasons and on the basis of the same information, two people can come to two different conclusions about what is good practice in a case. For example, families, social workers and their organisations often have very different thoughts on what to do in the field of child protection. The press and public opinion are often divided on how to protect children from abuse and neglect.

Even if they change in the long term, conceptions of good practice are usually quite stable in the short and medium term. So using the words of Reamer (2008, p.62), it is possible to say that *professional mistakes* occur 'when practitioners depart from widely accepted standards and best practices in the profession'. More specifically, Dillon (2003, pp.14–15) defines a mistake in clinical practice as 'an attitude, behaviour, feeling, response, communication, contextual arrangement, or strategy for work that undermines the stated purpose or specific interest of a given intervention'.

In case of a negative outcome, the most important question to decide is whether this is a case of a professional mistake or not: Was the *decision* leading to the mistake *defensible and reasonable*? A decision can be classified as defensible when a responsible body of co-professionals would have made the same decision in the same circumstances (Carson 1996), that is when an accredited methodology has been used and the decision has been shared or could have been shared with colleagues (Kemshall 2001).

Following appropriate methodologies, social workers operate to improve the conditions of their service users but unexpected worsening of the situation may happen in the form of a complication of the situation without an error having occurred. At the same time, many errors have no negative consequences because they have a limited impact on the situation or are recognised before harm occurs.

The other side of error prevention systems and risk management

Recognising mistakes before they happen and before harm occurs is the most important function of *error prevention systems*. A growing number of organisations are developing structures and strategies to prevent error and manage risk in energy and industrial fields but also, more recently, in health and social care, especially in hospitals and similar institutions. The more complex the field (and human beings are definitely very complex), the more the *risk* is a constant reality. In general, the latter can be defined as 'a decision-making situation where the outcomes are uncertain and where benefits are sought but undesirable outcomes are possible' (Taylor 2013, p.10).

Risk is deeply connected to the concept of *latent error*: there are 'active errors, whose effects are felt almost immediately, and latent errors whose adverse consequences may lie dormant within the system for a long time, only becoming evident when they combine with other factors to breach the system's defences' (Reason 1990, p.173). Latent errors can lead to tragic outcomes if combined with other factors so paying attention to sentinel events or minor mistakes is the most effective strategy in preventing graver errors. When latent errors are detected, systemic or organisational changes may be taken not only to avert risks but also to bring general improvements to individuals and organisations. Ignoring the existence of latent errors would be as silly as dismissing the low level of the fuel gauge and continuing to drive because you think there is no time to stop and fill the tank (Sicora 2017).

According to Schulz (2010), organisational error prevention systems should be based on the following *central principles* to be really effective: *acceptance of the likelihood of error*, open and democratic communication and reliance on verifiable data. It is hard to admit something went wrong because everyone wants to avoid blame and shame. Even if everybody would agree with sentences like 'to err is human' and 'everyone makes mistakes', most people tend to consider them acceptable for the others not for themselves. But, if the first signs of a mistake are denied or undervalued and not sufficiently considered it is likely that no action is taken to repair or limit negative impacts and harm before they become really unsustainable.

It could be easier to say 'I am wrong' if there was a wider acceptance of the likelihood of error; of course not in terms of laxity or irresponsibility. Furthermore, sometimes the effects of shame become a real and serious problem for many people: based on experiences in Health Service Accident and Emergency Departments, Sanders, Pattison, and Hurwitz (2011) found out that nurses and other practitioners may prefer not to reveal their mistakes, or may even try to lie or deceive others in order to avoid shame and hide their own sense of inadequacy. Denial of mistakes can be very dangerous when it prevents taking action in order to repair or reduce their negative outcomes. The effect of social workers' shame on their well-being is so pervasive in many contexts that the construction of shame-sensitive organisations and shame-resilient practitioners is vital to reduce the impact of this feeling on the quality of the services users receive (Gibson 2014).

Being wrong is an emotional experience. It implies not only the recognition of a deviation from external reality and an internal change in what the subject believes and his/her consequent acts, but also the condition of being stuck in wrongness with no immediate way out (Schulz 2010). This is unpleasant, especially when accompanied by the sight of the damage done and when internal or external voices not only blame for the wrong action but also criticise the whole person. The shift from 'I/you made a mistake' to 'I am/You are a failure', that is 'I am/you are a failure as a practitioner or even as a person' is easy and common and shame may be the resulting feeling. Even if criticism may be useful feedback to give constructive opportunities of learning from mistakes, it is more often felt by people as an attack and a sabotage to their own self-confidence and this produces more commonly a defensive reaction aimed at avoiding shame rather than listening and reflecting. In these circumstances, learning from mistakes becomes almost impossible (Sicora 2017). Shame and its counterpart, that is recognition, are both concepts that influence social work practice deeply and are experienced by both social workers and their service users (Frost 2016).

The acceptance of the likelihood of error makes it easier to depower shame and feelings of inadequacy but also implicates the recognition that there is not such a thing like an error-free activity. At the same time, any adverse result is always the result of the actions and interactions of many subjects.

The so-called 'Swiss cheese model' described by Reason (1990) helps to better understand this concept and see its connections with the need of *open communication within organisations in order to circulate reliable, verifiable, and accurate data* on the processes leading to mistakes. Adverse events are the results of intricate chains of events always involving more than a single individual. Complex systems can be represented as a set of layers, one behind the other as shown in Figure 1. These are:

(1) decision-makers (for example, policy-makers);
(2) line management (related to the implementation of the strategies decided at the previous level);
(3) preconditions (environmental conditions, codes of practice, physical and psychological conditions, skills, knowledge and motivation of workers, etc.);
(4) productive activities (in terms of services, as well as goods);
(5) defences (any safeguards against foreseeable hazards).

These layers may have one or more 'holes', which represent fallible decisions, deficiencies or unsafe acts. Only if all the layers have 'holes' on the same line the route of potential mistake continues till its occurrence. None is guilty, but everybody has a part of responsibility when negative outcomes occur. Looking for scapegoats and removing them from their job is easy but not an effective solution. They are even dangerous because they give the illusion that security has been obtained and consequently there is no need of further actions and defences.

The last layer is even more important because in most of the systems it is unlikely the previous layers are entirely intact and without holes. It is clear that, as every human being, policy-makers and managers are not perfect. And, at the same time, it is impossible to find workers who are completely skilled, in ideal conditions of no stress and in possession of all the knowledge required for their job. So it is important to create some defences, like, for example, a colleague reading and double checking a report

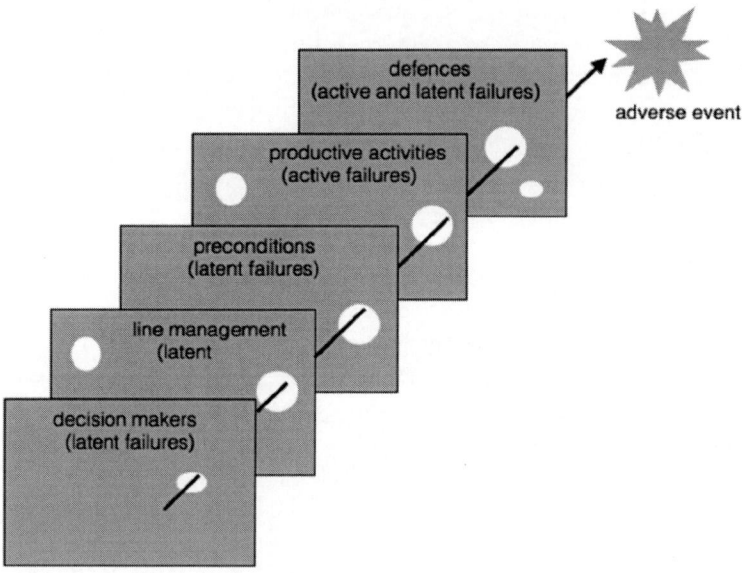

FIGURE 1 Reason's Swiss cheese model (Adapted from Reason 1990).

before sending it to the authority that has to decide on sensitive cases, especially when the practitioner is new in that service and without so much experience. But people in different layers often ignored the conditions of the others. Most of the times they see the 'holes' closer to them but not the breaches in the others and it is even more unlikely they are aware of the alignment existing in the system. This is the reason why feedbacks between layers are the prerequisite to any rapid and effective response aimed at reducing the risk of a bad outcome. Feedback loops, like reporting accidents and audits, and well-chosen and measured indicators may increase safety considerably in any technological system (Reason 1990). Social work organisations function this way as well and also here many major mistakes happen when people do not share information and knowledge horizontally (amongst colleagues) and vertically (between management and workers).

Balancing safety and production goals is another important category of deci-sion-making in many fields. Talking mostly about industrial processes, Reason (1990, p.203) states that 'all organisations have to allocate resources to two distinct goals: pro-duction and safety. In the long term, these are clearly compatible goals. But, given that all resources are finite, there are likely to be many occasions on which there are short-term conflicts of interest. Resources allocated to the pursuit of production could diminish those available for safety; the converse is also true'. Translating 'production' into service users' well-being, things do not seem much different also in social work: for example, when the ratio between social workers and service users is high, the first have more time to take care of the second and this, at parity of other conditions, leads to more precise assessment and more effective planning and intervention. In these fa-vourable conditions mistakes are less likely to occur. But reality is different and shortage of time is very common in most of health and social services. Moreover, safety at any cost may produce paradoxically more risk. Data from the field of medicine are sadly remarkable: the fact that doctors order tests and treatment to avoid the risk of wrong assessments and unfair prosecution because of omissions or mistakes has huge monetary and human costs. A recent study in the USA estimates that radiation from computed tomography could cause 1.5–2.0% of all cancers and 92.5% of surgeons declare they have ordered imaging tests to protect themselves from lawsuits (Hettrich et al. 2010). The same risk aversion be at the origin of some negative outcome in social work, for example, when children are taken away from their families to avoid any risk of abuse and maltreatment or, on the contrary, when children are kept in their families to avoid the risk of traumatic removal or strong reaction from their parents. Moreover, using the outcomes of an ethnographic study in some areas of England and Wales on the implementation of IT systems, generically known as the Integrated Children's System (ICS), Broadhurst et al. (2010) demonstrates that current attempts to increase safety in child welfare practices, through standardised procedures and micro-manage decisions, may have paradoxically the contrary effect and subtract time and energy to support families.

All this leads to the dilemma on the limits of any process based on the principle of 'trial and error': When is it acceptable to try something new (and, in some cases, a bit risky) if ordinary and normal strategies were tried and failed? How far social workers can go in term of exploration and experimentation? How is it possible to make effective intervention applying general rules and theoretical principles to situations that in social work are often unique and unrepeatable?

However, social workers have *ethical ties and responsibilities towards* their *service users* and so cannot afford to make damaging mistakes. Decision-making needs to be defensible and reasonable (a professional methodology and shared communication with colleagues are basic requirements for this) and is improved by reflective service users and their active contribution. In fact, the involvement of the latter in social work decisions and interventions makes easier to obtain the expected and agreed objectives and reduces the risks of mistakes. This *cooperative approach* brings to mind Schön's concept of the reflective client (Schön 1983) in social work and is in tune with the idea of service users as 'experts by experience'.

The 'need' to search for new ideas and solutions in difficult situations is clear, as well as that proceeding by 'trial and error' when the usual paths are not working has specific ethical limits and must be always conducted in the supreme interest of the service users, first of all the present ones but also those in the future, who will benefit from the actions of a more skilful practitioner.

Ethical dilemmas are common in social work and, in many situations, the borderline between what is right and what is wrong is quite controversial. For example, does the safety older people find in a retirement home come first or the warmth and the familiarity they have in their own houses? Is the autonomy of homeless people who refuse to access homeless shelters more important than the safety considered best by the society they live in? Throughout the world, *codes of ethics* help and guide social workers in answering these and other similar questions and to reduce harm and risks for service users when ethical dilemmas and conflicts of interests arise. Some of these documents also highlight the importance of reflection and constructive criticism amongst colleagues as a mutual support in decision-making processes (Sicora 2017).

Reflective tools and strategies

Reflective practice is considered the most effective strategy in social work, education, nursing and other disciplines within the health and social professions because it helps workers to learn from their experience and develop their professional knowledge and skills in a never-ending process (amongst many, see, Bolton 2010; Bruce 2013; Bulman 2004; Fook, White, & Gardner 2006; Ingram, Fenton, Hodson, & Jindal-Snape 2014; Ruch 2009; Taylor 2010; Thompson & Thompson 2008; and others). At the end of a working day everybody reflects on what happened, sometimes even too much since it is not easy to abandon the many thoughts and questions arising from the events of the day, especially if something unexpected occurs: Why did it happen, this and that? What is the meaning of this? Where this will take me? What went wrong?

In daily life and in scientific research reflection and discovery is most of all a matter of questions. Skilled practitioners have no right answers for everything but have the right questions that can guide the search for the meanings of daily practice and the directions for effective actions. Questions, reflective frameworks and writing are some of the most effective tools in reflective practice. Reflective friends and the involvement of organisations are some of the most successful strategies.

Questions are the key instrument of any reflection process. The smarter they are the better and deeper the exploration is. A smart question is something that puzzles and makes people say 'this is really a good question!' and start going to the bottom of the issue and looking for an answer. At the same time, 'smart' questions are capable of generating knowledge because they guide the search towards the answers and help to explore unknown areas that previously were not considered and where solutions for problems may be found. As the poet and philosopher Solomon Ibn Gabirol said (Johnson 2003, p.158) 'a wise man's question contains half the answer'.

Practitioners may formulate 'smart questions' or they may use reflective frameworks that consist of sets of predefined questions. There are many of them in the literature and they can be simple, with a very few questions, or complex, with long list of questions scanning in details any aspect of the episode under investigation (Sicora 2017). The simplest and more successful of these reflective frameworks is probably the three Borton's questions 'what', 'so what', 'now what' (Borton 1970) generating more specific questions like, for example (Rolfe, Freshwater, & Jasper 2001):

- What is the problem? What did I do? What were the consequences for the user?
- So what does the event teach me? So what could I have done to make it better?
- Now what do I have to do to make things better? Now what do I have to do to feel better?

More complex reflective frameworks, for example the Gibbs' reflective cycle (1988), stimulate similar mental operations. They recall in detail what happens (also in term of emotions) and help to see the negative and positive in the episode. In fact, the most clear success has always something 'bad' and even the graver failure produces something 'good' like, for example, a strong pressure to learn and act to do better in the future). Moreover, these reflective frameworks make easier to understand the interaction of elements behind the appearance of what happened and learn what to do differently if a similar case occurs.

Combining some of the concepts and ideas above (especially from the Gibbs' reflective cycle), a reflective framework focused on errors and failures has been developed to help social workers to go deeper in the understanding of their failures and mistakes (Sicora 2017). The following reduced version may help to conduct the reflection process more quickly (the full version has more than 91 questions) focusing the attention on the most important points.

1. DESCRIPTION

1.1. What happened, where and when? Who was involved? Where were you? Who else was with you? Why were you there? Were these normal/normative circumstances?

1.2. Which part in what happened did you undertake? Which part did the others undertake? What was your role in the event and what was the role of each of the others?

2. FEELINGS

2.1. How did you feel, that is, what were your emotions (positive and negative) and thoughts?

2.2. What did the other people involved in the event do, think and feel? How do you know this?

3. ASSESSMENT

3.1. What would you describe as positive and what might be described as negative in the experience?

3.2. What do you think specifically went wrong? For whom? According to which technical ideas or ethical principles?

4. ANALYSIS

4.1. Why did you behave like you did?

4.2. What chain of events led to the error/failure? What was the role of each of the following stages/levels?

4.2.1. top level decision-makers (social policies, direction, goal of general and inherent resource allocation);

4.2.2. line management (i.e. implementation by the executive level of the strategies defined at the above level);

4.2.3. preconditions (motivations, equipment, etc.) of the subjects and factors directly involved in the implementation of social work services such as users, practitioners, material resources, etc.;

4.2.4. productive activities (when the analysed event occurred);

4.2.5. defence systems (amongst the issues to be included there are supervision, peers cooperation amongst colleagues and others).

5. CONCLUSION

5.1. What factors caused the error/failure to happen? Which are the three most important factors?

5.2. If you could go back in time, what would you do differently?

6. ACTION PLAN

6.1. What do you need to change? What can you do differently next time when you deal with a similar case?

6.2. What do you need to work on and how will you work on it?

Reflective frameworks are helpful at an individual level and in cooperation with other people, like during face-to-face interactions with a colleague or in team discussions. Having a 'critical friend' who listens and assists in making some sense of relevant episodes is particularly useful. Critical friends provide the necessary support and stimulation for their colleagues by asking relevant and 'smart' questions, giving supportive comments and suggestions on seeing things from different perspectives. Professional respect and confidentiality are two basic requirements when one plays this role (Taylor 2010).

Reflection can be carried out as a dialogue, interior or with an interlocutor, also in written form. Sheets of paper and computer screens become mirrors to grasp aspects and meanings lost using other strategies and tools. Reflective writing, in its essence, is the deliberate use of strategies of writing as a way of reflecting and learning from experience. When characterised by objectivity and the attempt to stand back from the considered events, it leads to analytical and 'rational' insight. On the other hand, the creative use of imagination and metaphors helps to express emotions and enter in contact with other forms of knowledge, not only on the episode but also on the whole self of the practitioner. Since mistakes and failures often produce strong feelings and emotions, reflective writing works very well in expressing and elaborating the latter.

An example of the first form of writing (more analytical and rational) is the use of the above reflective framework or other structured similar tools. Other examples of this kind are: critical incident analysis, dialogical writing (creating a conversation through questions and answers), creating an on-going record, SWOT analysis (identifying the strengths, weaknesses, opportunities and threats within an experience), identifying three-a-day (for example, 'Three things I have learned today are …'), page-a-day record of experiences. On the other hand, there are also several forms of creative strategies like: writing an unsent letter or email, to a nominated other person (for example, a close friend) or as the other person, or as a journalist, or writing poetry, a story or a review in a particular style, like fantasy, science-fiction and so on (Jasper 2004; and Rolfe et al. 2001).

It is evident that social workers do not have much time to write their reflections. For this reason, strategies of concise reflective writing (that is with a limited number of words and/or characters) are especially useful because they produce very rich material that can give a global view on what happened and, especially if stored weeks after weeks, is not too much influenced by the last episodes and the moment when the final reflection is carried out.

The following three examples of narratives reduced to 160 characters show how to use extreme concise reflective writing at the end of a more detailed process of reflection (for example, after answering all the questions of a reflective framework mentally or verbally) in order to highlight what mistakes and event occurred at the workplace teach (Sicora 2017, p.152):

> Elder found dead 20 days later because neighbours gave the alarm. Social worker didn't do what she had to do. Never be superficial in apparently easy cases.

> Teenager in community unable to return home but against any fostering. I didn't insist. He returned to his addicted mother and he also became so. I have to be more determined!

> Difficult interview. I do not like these relatives. It's useless. They do not understand. Maybe they did not listen. Maybe I have to. Well, next time I will.

Conclusion: a never-ending process impossible to complete?

Mistakes are impossible to eradicate but their negative impact and the likelihood of their recurrence can be reduced. In pursuing these goals, learning from mistakes and first of all being aware of them, is vital and may help social workers to become more skilled and effective in their job. Reflection on mistakes is technically possible (using, for example, the structured tools and strategies mentioned before) and ethically desirable because it reduces the harm social work occasionally may cause. On the other hand, extreme risk aversion may paradoxically lead to increases in other forms of risk and prevent the search for innovative solutions to problems that cannot be solved with traditional methods.

The acceptance of the likelihood of error does not mean to grant a licence to make irresponsible mistakes. On the contrary, an honest and frank reflection on their experiences helps social workers to detect latent errors in their behaviour and in their organisations and prevent the worst mistakes. It is by no means a way to loosen the essential and unavoidable ethical ties and responsibilities towards service users, but it may strengthen the cooperation with the latter and help to find new ways to make social work stronger and more effective.

ORCID

Alessandro Sicora 🆔 http://orcid.org/0000-0002-7944-8144

References

Bolton, G. (2010). *Reflective practice: Writing and professional development* (3rd ed.). London: Sage.

Borton, T. (1970). *Reach, touch and teach*. New York, NY: McGraw-Hill.

Broadhurst, K., Wastell, D., White, S., Hall, C., Peckover, S., Thompson, K., … Davey, D. (2010). Performing 'initial assessment': Identifying the latent conditions for error at the front-door of local authority children's services. *British Journal of Social Work, 40*(2), 352–370. doi:10.1093/bjsw/bcn162

Bruce, L. (2013). *Reflective practice for social workers: A handbook for developing professional confidence*. Maidenhead: Open University Press.

Bulman, C. (2004). An introduction to reflection. In C. Bulman & S. Schutz (Eds.), *Reflective practice in nursing* (3rd ed., pp. 1–24). London: Blackwell.

Carson, D. (1996). Risking legal repercussions. In H. Kemshall & L. Pritchard (Eds.), *Good practice in risk assessment and management* (Vol. 1, pp. 3–12). London: Jessica Kingsley.

Dillon, C. (2003). *Learning from mistakes in clinical practice*. Belmont, CA: Brooks/Cole.

Fook, J., White, S., & Gardner, F. (2006). Critical reflection: A review of contemporary literature and understanding. In S. White, J. Fook, & F. Gardner (Eds.), *Critical reflection in health and social care* (pp. 3–20). Berkshire: Open University Press.

Frost, L. (2016). Exploring the concepts of recognition and shame for social work. *Journal of Social Work Practice, 30*(4), 431–446. doi:10.1080/02650533.2015.1132689

Gibbs, G. (1988). *Learning by doing: A guide to teaching and learning methods*. London: Further Education Unit.

Gibson, M. (2014). Social worker shame in child and family social work: Inadequacy, failure, and the struggle to practise humanely. *Journal of Social Work Practice, 28*(4), 417–431. doi:10.1080/02650533.2014.913237

Hettrich, C. M., Mather, R. C., Sethi, M. K., Nunley, R. M., Jahangir, A. A., & the Washington Health Policy Fellows. (2010, December 8–10). The costs of defensive medicine. *AAOS Now*.

Ingram, R., Fenton, J., Hodson, A., & Jindal-Snape, D. (2014). *Reflective social work practice*. Basingstoke: Palgrave.

International Association of Social Workers, & International Association of School of Social Work. (2014). Global definition of social work. Retrieved from http://ifsw.org/get-involved/global-definition-of-social-work/

Jasper, M. (2004). Using journals and diaries within reflective practice. In C. Bulman & S. Schutz (Eds.), *Reflective practice in nursing* (3rd ed., pp. 94–112). London: Blackwell.

Johnson, L. A. (2003). *A toolbox for humanity: 3000 years of thought*. Victoria: Trafford.

Kemshall, H. (2001). *Risk assessment and management of known sexual and violent offenders: A review of current issues*. London: Crown.

Reamer, F. G. (2008). Social workers' management of error: Ethical and risk management issues. *Families in Society: The Journal of Contemporary Social Services, 89*(1), 61–68. doi:10.1606/1044-3894.3710

Reason, J. (1990). *Human error*. Cambridge: Cambridge University Press.

Rolfe, G., Freshwater, D., & Jasper, M. (2001). *Critical reflection for nursing and the helping professions: A users guide*. Basingstoke: Palgrave.

Ruch, G. (2009). *Post-qualifying child care social work: Developing reflective practice*. London: Sage.

Sanders, K., Pattison, S., & Hurwitz, B. (2011). Tracking shame and humiliation in accident and emergency. *Nursing Philosophy, 12*, 83–93.

Schön, D. A. (1983). *The reflective practitioner: How professionals think in action*. New York, NY: Basic Books.

Schulz, K. (2010). *Being wrong: Adventures in the margin of error*. New York, NY: HarperCollins.

Sicora, A. (2017). *Reflective practice and learning from mistakes in social work*. Bristol: Policy Press.

Taylor, B. J. (2010). *Reflective practice for healthcare professionals* (3rd ed.). Berkshire: McGraw-Hill.

Taylor, B. J. (2013). *Professional decision making and risk in social work* (2nd ed.). London: Sage.

Thompson, S., & Thompson, N. (2008). *The critically reflective practitioner*. New York, NY: Palgrave Macmillan.

Index